Mikael D.Z. Kimelman, F

GROUP TREATMENT OF NEUROGENIC

COMMUNICATION DISORDERS

GROUP TREATMENT OF NEUROGENIC COMMUNICATION DISORDERS

The Expert Clinician's Approach

Edited by

Roberta J. Elman, Ph.D., CCC-SLP, BC-NCD

President and Founder, Aphasia Center of California, Oakland

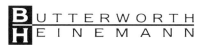

Boston   Oxford   Johannesburg   Melbourne   New Delhi   Singapore

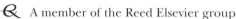

Library of Congress Cataloging-in-Publication Data

Group treatment of neurogenic communication disorders : the expert clinician's approach/edited by Roberta J. Elman.
      p.   cm.
    Includes bibliographical references and index.
    ISBN 0-7506-9084-4
    1. Aphasic persons--Rehabilitation. 2. Group speech therapy.
3. Articulation disorders--Patients--Rehabilitation. 4. Brain
damage--Patients--Rehabilitation. I. Elman, Roberta J.
    [DNLM: 1. Aphasia--rehabilitation. 2. Communication Disorders-
-rehabilitation. 3. Psychotherapy, Group. WL 340.5G882 1999]
RC425.G76 1999
616.85'5206--dc21
DNLM/DLC
for Library of Congress   98-35192
                                          CIP

British Library Cataloguing in Publication Data
A catalogue record for this book is available from the British Library.

The publisher offers special discounts on bulk orders of this book.
For information, please contact:
Manager of Special Sales
Butterworth–Heinemann
225 Wildwood Avenue
Woburn, MA 01801-2041
Tel: 781-904-2500
Fax: 781-904-2620

For information on all Butterworth–Heinemann publications available, contact our World Wide Web home page at: http://www.bh.com

10 9 8 7 6 5 4 3 2 1

Printed in the United States of America

Never doubt that a small group of thoughtful,
committed people can change the world.
Indeed, it is the only thing that ever has.
—Margaret Mead

Contents

SECTION V: MOTOR SPEECH DISORDERS

Contributing Authors

Pelagie M. Beeson, Ph.D., CCC-SLP, BC-NCD
Assistant Research Scientist, National Center for Neurogenic Communication Disorders and Department of Speech and Hearing Sciences, University of Arizona, Tucson

Ellen Bernstein-Ellis, M.A., CCC-SLP
Speech-Language Pathologist, Aphasia Center of California, Oakland

Mary Boyle, Ph.D., CCC-SLP, BC-NCD
Director, Speech-Language and Audiology Department, The Winifred Masterson Burke Rehabilitation Hospital, White Plains, New York

Cynthia Busch, Ph.D., CCC-SLP
Speech-Language Pathology Consultant to Medicare for Blue Cross and Blue Shield of Minnesota; Part-time Instructor in Communication Disorders, University of Minnesota, Minneapolis, and Mankato State University, Mankato, Minnesota

Leora R. Cherney, Ph.D., CCC-SLP, BC-NCD
Associate Professor of Physical Medicine and Rehabilitation, Northwestern University Medical School, Chicago; Clinical Educator and Researcher, Center for Clinical Excellence, Rehabilitation Institute of Chicago

Rochelle Cohen-Schneider, B.A., CASLPO
Program Coordinator, Pat Arato Aphasia Centre, Toronto

Ruth Coles, M.Sc., MRCSLT
Director, Action for Dysphasic Adults, London

Sandra Curtis, M.A., CCC-SLP
Research Coordinator, The Aphasia Center, Texas Woman's University, Dallas

Christine Eales, M.Sc., MRCSLT
Regional Development Advisor, Action for Dysphasic Adults, London; Rivermead Rehabilitation Centre, Oxford, United Kingdom

Gayle J. Ellis, M.A., CCC-SLP
Area Manager, RehabVisions, Omaha, Nebraska

Roberta J. Elman, Ph.D., CCC-SLP, BC-NCD
President and Founder, Aphasia Center of California, Oakland

Susan E. Adair Ewing, M.A., CCC-SLP
Speech-Language Pathologist, Aphasia Center of California, Oakland

Jean Ford, Ph.D., CCC-SLP
Director, The Aphasia Center, Texas Woman's University, Dallas; Assistant Clinical Professor of Communication Sciences and Disorders, Texas Woman's University, Dallas

Kathryn L. Garrett, Ph.D., CCC-SLP
Assistant Professor of Speech-Language Pathology, Duquesne University, Pittsburgh

Rita J. Gillis, Ph.D., CCC-SLP
Independent Consultant in Rehabilitation, Gulf Breeze, Florida

Marjorie A. Graham, M.S., CCC-SLP
Director, Faxton Hospital Hearing and Speech Center, Utica, New York

Christina V. Green, M.A., CCC-SLP
Speech-Language Pathologist, Eddy Cohoes Rehabilitation Center, Cohoes, New York

Anita S. Halper, M.A., CCC-SLP, BC-NCD
Associate Professor of Physical Medicine and Rehabilitation and Clinical Associate Professor of Communication Sciences and Disorders, Northwestern University Medical School, Chicago; Project Support Specialist, Rehabilitation Institute of Chicago

Audrey L. Holland, Ph.D., CCC-SLP, BC-NCD
Professor, Department of Speech and Hearing Sciences and National Center for Neurogenic Communication Disorders, University of Arizona, Tucson

Aura Kagan, M.A., CASLPO
Program and Research Director, Pat Arato Aphasia Centre, Toronto

Ann Marie Marchese, M.S., CCC-SLP
Clinical Education Coordinator, Speech-Language and Audiology Department, The Winifred Masterson Burke Rehabilitation Hospital, White Plains, New York

Robert C. Marshall, Ph.D., CCC-SLP, BC-NCD
Associate Professor, Department of Communicative Disorders, University of Rhode Island, Kingston

Roger Ross, MIA
Publishing Consultant, Scottsdale, Arizona

Patricia Smith, M.S., PT-NCS
Assistant Professor of Physical Therapy, University of Texas Southwestern Medical Center, Dallas

Delaina Walker-Batson, Ph.D., CCC-SLP
Professor of Communication Sciences, The Aphasia Center, Texas Woman's University, Dallas; Associate Clinical Professor of Neurology and Radiology, University of Texas Southwestern Medical Center, Dallas

Preface

Group treatment is enjoying a renaissance. Given the significant changes to health care systems throughout the world, many clinicians are searching for different ways to treat individuals who have neurogenic communication disorders. Many clinicians are frustrated by the reductions in authorized individual treatment now provided for their clients. Many are also frustrated by the lack of generalization of meaningful treatment gains to the client's home or other outside environments. These frustrations have a silver lining, however: Clinicians are considering group treatment as a possible solution to the restrictions currently associated with one-to-one treatment.

My introduction to group treatment occurred in 1989 on a visit to the Aphasia Centre—North York (now the Pat Arato Aphasia Centre). While observing the 15 or more groups in session that day, I was amazed by the dynamic interactions and variety of communication that surrounded me. Individuals with aphasia of all types and severities were communicating in ways that had never occurred in my one-to-one treatment sessions. Behaviors that I had been unable to teach or that had failed to generalize to outside environments were everywhere. I realized that the group environment provided many advantages over my small treatment room. This realization came before the impact of managed care on my clients' health care reimbursement. Regardless of funding, communication changes appeared to be happening in the groups that were not typical in one-to-one sessions. Since the fall of 1989, I have devoted the majority of my clinical and research time to investigating the benefits and efficacy of group communication treatment. The more I investigate, the more I am convinced. The statistical tests from an efficacy study we conducted confirmed what we were seeing with our own eyes and hearing from our clients and their families. Real-life communication change was occurring in those with chronic aphasia after only 2 months of group communication treatment. People were changing in ways that I never anticipated. People who had withdrawn from family and friends began to renew their ties. People who had been fearful to go out into the community began to use public transportation. People who had thought they were alone learned that others "walked in their shoes." For me, there was no turning back. The power of group treatment to effect meaningful change was clear.

I am convinced that group treatment is the silver lining in the often rather depressing world of our current health care system. However, the majority of speech-language pathologists do not receive training in conducting group treatment. Group dynamics are complex. If individual treatment can be compared to teaching a musical instrument, group treatment is much like conducting an orchestra. The clinician must keep in mind the communicative strengths and weaknesses of all group members. In addition, personality issues are overlaid, because group dynamics and group process are more than a sum of their individual parts. Although group treatment can be quite challenging, the potential rewards are well worth the efforts.

This book grew out of my realization that books on neurogenic communication disorders often did not make more than a passing reference to group treatment. Given the growing number of clinicians who are interested in group treatment, a book was needed that gave specific information about how the clinicians who were experienced in "doing" groups actually practiced. This book fills that need. I asked expert clinicians from the United States, Canada, and the United Kingdom to write chapters based on the programs in which they practiced. Clinical information was gathered on a range of exemplary group treatment programs for individuals with neurogenic communication disorders.

All of the chapters in this book are written by practicing expert clinicians. To ensure continuity, chapter authors were asked to use the following general outline, when applicable, to describe their programs: philosophy of program, entry criteria, client assessment, establishment of treatment goals, documentation of progress, clinical techniques used, discharge criteria, and reimbursement issues. In their own words, these clinicians provide detailed information on the day-to-day workings of their programs. Whenever possible, case examples and protocols for assessment or documentation are provided. It is hoped that the reader will acquire an excellent understanding of each specific group communication treatment program and begin to see similarities and differences among the programs. Just as there is no one "right" approach to living life, there is no one "right" approach to treating individuals with neurogenic communication disorders. It is hoped that as you read the following chapters, you will take from each what resonates loudest for you, your work setting, and most important, the individuals with whom you work.

The first four chapters provide general information regarding group treatment. In Chapter 1, I introduce the field of group treatment, including a rationale for conducting group treatment and a brief review of the studies that have investigated its efficacy. In Chapter 2, Susan E. Adair Ewing provides an overview of group process, group dynamics, and group techniques that need to be considered and understood for group treatment to be effective. This material is critical for conducting successful groups but is often absent in the speech-language pathology undergraduate or graduate curriculum. In Chapter 3, Kathryn L. Garrett offers suggestions for measuring group outcomes. This chapter includes a list of measures that might be used or adapted by practicing clinicians along the continuum of "real-life" clinical settings. In Chapter 4, Cynthia Busch shares information gained from her experience as a Medicare reviewer that clinicians must know to receive reimbursement for group treatment.

The remaining chapters are written by practicing clinicians about specific group treatment programs. Although the majority of these chapters provide examples of group programs that treat individuals with aphasia, readers interested in any communication disorder will find helpful insights and practices in all of the chapters. It is suggested that every chapter be read for the clinical wisdom and gems within, regardless of the clientele served by the programs.

Chapters 5–7 cover aphasia group treatment programs facilitated by speech-language pathologists. Chapter 5, by Marjorie A. Graham, demonstrates how treatment groups can be effective, even in a subacute setting. In Chapter 6,

Ellen Bernstein-Ellis and I describe the daily workings of our community-based outpatient treatment groups at the Aphasia Center of California. Chapter 7, by Robert C. Marshall, illustrates how those with mild aphasia benefit from problem-focused groups in a program initially based at a VA Medical Center.

Chapters 8–10 give examples of university programs that have aphasia groups facilitated by students. In Chapter 8, Delaina Walker-Batson, Sandra Curtis, Patricia Smith, and Jean Ford provide details on the Aphasia Center LifeLink© program developed at Texas Woman's University in Dallas. In Chapter 9, Audrey L. Holland and Pelagie M. Beeson offer the wisdom they have gained regarding aphasia groups while supervising the University of Arizona's student-facilitated program. Chapter 10, by Kathryn L. Garrett and Gayle J. Ellis, presents group-scaffolded thematic discourse activities, originally developed at the University of Nebraska.

Chapters 11–13 provide examples of aphasia groups that are volunteer based. In Chapter 11, Aura Kagan and Rochelle Cohen-Schneider describe their updated introductory program that is currently in use at the Pat Arato Aphasia Centre (formerly Aphasia Centre–North York). Chapter 12, by Ruth Coles and Christine Eales, provides an overview of the model program developed by the Action for Dysphasic Adults in the United Kingdom. In Chapter 13, Audrey L. Holland and Roger Ross discuss the benefits of group treatment from the viewpoint of someone living with aphasia.

In Chapter 14, Leora R. Cherney and Anita S. Halper discuss the variety of group treatment options for patients with right hemisphere damage. In Chapters 15 and 16, Rita J. Gillis provides a complete discussion of treatment issues and specific treatment groups used with individuals after traumatic brain injury. In Chapter 17, Mary Boyle, Ann Marie Marchese, and Christina V. Green describe group therapy for those with dysarthria.

This book can be used in classes and clinical practica for advanced undergraduates and graduate students in speech-language pathology. Clinicians who are interested in group treatment should find the information practical and easily applicable to a wide range of clients and settings. The information in this book should also prove of value to students and professionals in other heath-related disciplines.

RJE

Acknowledgments

The ideas and motivation leading to this book have evolved during the last 15 years. This book is but a snapshot in time.

I would like to thank two dear friends and colleagues who have added much to both my personal and professional growth. My trip to the Aphasia Centre–North York in 1989 was a true turning point. The visit changed my philosophy of what therapy should be and demonstrated many benefits of group treatment. This trip also resulted in an enduring friendship with Aura Kagan. Her enthusiasm for working with people with aphasia, coupled with her intellectual curiosity, have provided me with much inspiration to continue my evolution. Jon Lyon also has had a profound and lasting impact on my personal and professional life journey. Jon was responsible for introducing me to Aura and the Aphasia Centre–North York. His innovative approaches to conceptualizing and treating aphasia have influenced my overall treatment philosophy, as well as my daily clinical practice. In addition, thought-provoking discussions with Jon have been a catalyst for my continuing intellectual growth.

My Aphasia Center of California (ACC) colleagues, Ellen Bernstein-Ellis and Sue Ewing, have been instrumental in helping to create the ACC. Ellen and Sue have supported the vision that individuals with aphasia and their families need a place to receive group communication treatment for as long as it is desired. They have invested their intellect, their energy, and their time in making the ACC a reality.

Many others have shared their ideas, support, and friendship with me during the writing of this book and in the years preceding it. They include Sue Vanagas-Côté, Nina Simmons-Mackie, Eleanor Kalter, Tracy Cook, Mike Kimbarow, Carl Coehlo, JoAnn Lum, Mary Boyle, Audrey Holland, Jan Taylor, Cindy Thompson, Leora Cherney, Betty Bugaj, Esther Akiba, and Howard Banchefsky. These friends and colleagues, as well as many others, have helped to make my journey a rewarding and balanced one.

I would also like to acknowledge two former teachers who continue to serve as life-long role models: Bob Brookshire, who taught me that at times it is most important just to hold a patient's hand; and Carol Prutting, who shared her love of laughter, teaching, thinking, and life. I have also been fortunate to have had several teachers who tried to teach me how to write a sentence: Sandy Gerber, Jerry Siegel, and Terry Wertz. In my role as editor, their lessons continued.

These comments would not be complete without acknowledging those closest to me. They have provided their constant love, support, and encouragement throughout my career and especially during this project: my parents, Sid and Lil Elman, and my life partner, Steve Fry. They have been there to remind me of life's most important priorities.

And finally, my never-ending gratitude is extended to those with aphasia and their families. They are our ultimate teachers and most important audience.

SECTION I

Group Treatment— Fundamental and Professional Considerations

CHAPTER ONE

Introduction to Group Treatment of Neurogenic Communication Disorders

Roberta J. Elman

Traditional individual speech-language therapy focuses on didactic treatment tasks that strive to maximize linguistic and cognitive recovery [1–3]. In the clinical environment, traditional therapy tasks are typically chosen from language and cognitive modalities, such as speech production, spoken expression, auditory comprehension, reading, writing, attention, memory, organization, and problem solving. Treatment gains on targeted tasks are often observed, but generalization to functional communication, especially in real-life environments, has often been extremely difficult to achieve [4,5].

As reported in Elman and Bernstein-Ellis [6], group treatment for individuals with speech, language, or cognitive disorders may provide several advantages over individual treatment, especially for promoting generalization of functional communication to natural environments. There are several possible reasons for this: First, a group environment promotes interaction among members, which should foster pragmatic skills, including improved turn-taking and communicative initiation, as well as increasing the variety of communicative functions or speech acts [7,8]. In addition, the group environment provides the opportunity for a wider array of communicative partners and natural tasks, thereby increasing the likelihood that treatment gains will be generalized to home and community environments [9–12]. Second, group treatment may either directly or indirectly improve an individual's psychosocial functioning by providing a supportive environment in which communication is encouraged and modeled by the group facilitator and, perhaps more importantly, by the subject's peers [12–16]. Finally, group treatment is a cost-effective way of providing treatment to individuals compared to traditional individual speech-language therapy [10,17]. This is increasingly important as health care moves rapidly to a mature managed care model [18,19].

Kearns [10] provides a thorough review of the literature on group therapy for individuals with aphasia. Few publications address group communication treatment after traumatic brain injury, right hemisphere stroke, or motor speech disorders. This chapter presents a brief chronology of group treatment literature as a historic foundation for the chapters that follow. Emphasis is placed on studies that have investigated the efficacy of group communication treatment to provide clinicians with data that they can use to support group treatment. Authors of later chapters cite literature that is most relevant to their own treatment programs. The reader is also directed to other publications that present specific approaches to group treatment [20,21].

HISTORIC OVERVIEW OF GROUP TREATMENT FOR INDIVIDUALS WITH APHASIA

Until World War II, treatment for aphasia focused on individual didactic therapy. During and after the war, group treatment provided a practical solution for the large number of servicemen who needed speech-language services

[10]. Today, many see group aphasia treatment as an adjunct to individual therapy. Groups often focus on psychosocial adjustment and family counseling after stroke [22–24]. Fewer groups view improvement of communication skills as the central goal of the group. Of the published articles on group treatment for aphasia, most provide anecdotal accounts of treatment effectiveness [25–30]. Few studies address the question of treatment efficacy [6,17,31–33].

The reports of aphasia groups in the 1950s and the early 1960s focused on the communication benefit of groups [25–28]. In a description of group communication treatment for aphasia, Bloom stressed that patients should use and understand language in daily situations that are meaningful to them [27]. What may be surprising about these early anecdotal reports of group aphasia treatment is their focus on real-life activities. This focus seems to have been lost during the late 1960s and 1970s, probably due to the impact of behaviorism and the subsequent focus on stimulus-response treatment.

Child language research and treatment began to focus on pragmatics, or the use of language in context, in the 1970s [34–38]. This paradigm shift influenced adult language, and aphasiologists began to apply pragmatic principles to aphasia treatment in the 1980s [7,8,39–45]. During and after this time, several studies investigated the effectiveness of group communication treatment after stroke or brain injury.

EFFICACY OF GROUP COMMUNICATION TREATMENT

A 1982 group treatment study by Aten, Caligiuri, and Holland [17] tested whether functional communication treatment was effective for seven nonfluent, chronically aphasic patients who had not shown recent change on retesting with the Porch Index of Communicative Ability (PICA) [46] after "language-based" treatment. A formal control group or control condition was not used in this study. Group treatment was provided 2 hours weekly for 12 weeks and concentrated on improving functional communication in simulated real-life situations. These situations included activities such as shopping, giving and receiving directions, and reading labels and signs. Aten et al. measured significant improvement on the Communicative Abilities in Daily Living (CADL) test [47] but not in linguistic skills as measured by the PICA.

A partial replication of the Aten et al. study was provided by Bollinger, Musson, and Holland [31]. In this study, group treatment was provided using a treatment-withdrawal design, in which "structured" treatment was followed by a period of no treatment. Ten chronically aphasic individuals who were at least 18 months post-onset received 3 hours a week of group treatment for a total of 40 weeks. Ten-week segments of "contemporary group treatment" and "structured television-viewing group treatment" alternated with 10 weeks of no treatment. Contemporary group treatment consisted of greetings and socialization, a core activity focusing on a real-life activity, and specific communication-related activities, such as group repetition of words and naming activities. Structured television-viewing group treatment consisted of subjects watching selected television programs for later group discussion of certain communicative elements. Bollinger et al. found significant improvement on both the CADL and the PICA but not on the Auditory Comprehension Test for Sentences [48]. Results did not demonstrate either treatment to be superior.

Wertz and colleagues [32] give an important empiric account of the efficacy of group treatment for aphasia. The purpose of their study was to compare individual treatment to group treatment. Using random assignment, aphasic subjects received 8 hours of either individual or group treatment weekly. Group treatment consisted of general discussions of current events or other topics and did not include direct manipulation of linguistic skills. In contrast to Aten et al. [17] or Bollinger et al. [31], group treatment did not focus on real-life situations for communication. Wertz and colleagues found that the PICA was the only measure that showed significant differences between individual and group treatment. No significant differences were apparent on the other language tests. Wertz et al. state, "Our results indicate that individual treatment may be slightly superior to group treatment. However, the improvement displayed by our group-treated patients and the cost-effective advantages of group therapy should prompt speech-language pathologists to consider it for at least part of an aphasic patient's care" [32].

Elman and Bernstein-Ellis [6,33] examined the effect of group communication treatment on the linguistic and communicative performance of adults with chronic aphasia. This study was the first to control for social contact. Subjects were randomly assigned to two immediate-treatment and two deferred-treatment groups, which were balanced for age, education level, and initial aphasia severity. Twenty-four subjects completed 4 months of treatment. All subjects received 5 hours per week of group communication treatment provided by a speech-language pathologist. Group communication treatment included increasing initiation of conversation and exchanging information using whatever communicative means possible. While awaiting group communication treatment, subjects in the deferred-treatment groups engaged in activities such as support, performance, or movement groups to control for possible effects of social contact. Linguistic and communication-dependent measures were administered to all subjects at entry, after 2 and 4 months of treatment, and after 4–6 weeks of no treatment. Results revealed that group communication treatment was effective. Deferred-treatment groups did not change significantly with social contact alone. Subjects receiving group communication treatment had significantly higher scores on communicative and linguistic measures than did subjects not receiving treatment. In addition, treatment benefits continued over time: Significant improvement occurred after 2 and 4 months of treatment. No significant decline in linguistic or communicative performance occurred at follow-up, approximately 6 weeks after group communication treatment ended.

Taken together, these studies strongly support the conclusion that group communication treatment is effective for individuals with aphasia. The following studies investigated the effectiveness of a group treatment program and a day treatment program for those with chronic traumatic brain injury.

Ehrlich and Sipes [49] reported on a group intervention program designed to improve the communication skills of those with traumatic brain injury. Six clients ranging in age from 18 to 42 who were 1 year or more postinjury participated in the treatment program. Subjects received 3 hours of treatment weekly over 12 weeks. Therapists acted as group facilitators, with clients expected to participate as both speakers and listeners. Giving feedback to other members regarding "on-task" behaviors was a focus of the treatment. Specific pragmatic behaviors were selected and targeted using role playing, videotaping of role playing, and evaluation of observed behaviors. A behavioral rating scale adapted from the Prutting and Kirchner protocol [38] was completed before and after treatment. Comparison of pre- and post-treatment scores was significant. Most improvement occurred in the area of topic maintenance, initiation of conversation, syntax, cohesiveness, and repair.

Ruff and Niemann [50] compared the efficacy of day treatment to computerized cognitive remediation. Twenty-four patients, all between 1 and 7 years after injury, were randomly assigned to one of the two treatment conditions. All subjects received treatment 4 days a week over an 8-week period. The authors considered day treatment the control condition. The day treatment condition consisted of 1 hour of morning group therapy followed by treatment focused on psychosocial functioning and activities of daily living. A 20- to 30-minute wrap-up group session finished each day. The computerized cognitive remediation condition consisted of structured cognitive retraining on the following cognitive modules: attention, visuospatial abilities, learning and memory, and problem solving. In addition to the computerized modules, patients in the cognitive remediation condition received the same daily morning and wrap-up group therapy sessions. Few significant differences were found between the two treatment conditions. Subjects in both treatments displayed a reduction in depression on the primary dependent variable, the Katz Adjustment Scale [51]. Ruff and Niemann concluded that ongoing structured activities, such as those found in a day treatment program, are beneficial for those with traumatic brain injuries, and the authors believe that such activities facilitate emotional and psychosocial adjustment.

FUTURE DIRECTIONS

It is surprising that so few empiric research studies have investigated the efficacy of group treatment for individuals with communication disorders. A literature search failed to find published research on the effectiveness of group communication treatment for those with either right hemisphere or motor speech disorders. On a daily basis, speech-language pathologists are asked to achieve functional communication improvement by their clients, the community, and third-party payers. Historically, this has been difficult to achieve using individual speech-language treatment. In his review of group therapy for aphasia, Kearns [10] states that we must overcome the incorrect assumption that group therapy has already been validated, and he strongly calls for further research. More data must be collected; our work is not yet done.

What is encouraging about the research done to date is the growing consensus that group communication treatment holds real promise as a treatment method. Given the rapidly changing health care reimbursement environment, including the emergence and dominance of a managed care model, group communication treatment for individuals appears to provide an effective and economical option for delivering neurogenic communication treatment.

REFERENCES

1. Davis A, Wilcox M. Adult Aphasia Rehabilitation. San Diego: College Hill Press, 1985.
2. Rosenbek J, LaPointe L, Wertz R. Aphasia: A Clinical Approach. Boston: College Hill Press, 1989.
3. Sarno M. Acquired Aphasia. San Diego: Academic, 1991.
4. Kearns K. Methodologies for Studying Generalization. In J Spradlin, L McReynolds (eds), Generalization Strategies in Communication Disorders. Toronto: BC Decker, 1989.
5. Thompson C. Generalization research in aphasia: a review of the literature. Clin Aphasiol 1989;18:195–222.
6. Elman RJ, Bernstein-Ellis EG. The efficacy of group communication treatment in adults with chronic aphasia. J Speech Lang Hear Res. (In press.)
7. Davis GA. Pragmatics and Treatment. In R Chapey (ed), Language Intervention Strategies in Adult Aphasia. Baltimore: Williams & Wilkins, 1986:251–265.
8. Wilcox M. Aphasia: pragmatic considerations. Top Lang Disord 1983;3:35–48.
9. Green G. Assessment and treatment of the adult with severe aphasia: aiming for functional generalisation. Aust J Hum Commun Disord 1982;10:11–23.
10. Kearns K. Group Therapy for Aphasia: Theoretical and Practical Considerations. In R Chapey (ed), Language Intervention Strategies in Adult Aphasia (3rd ed). Baltimore: Williams & Wilkins, 1994;304–321.
11. Lyon JG. Communicative use and participation in life for aphasic adults in natural settings: the scope of the problem. Am J Speech Lang Path 1992;1:7–14.
12. Lyon JG. Optimizing Communication and Participation in Life for Aphasic Adults and Their Primary Caregivers in Natural Settings: A Use Model for Treatment. In GL Wallace (ed), Adult Aphasia Rehabilitation. Boston: Butterworth–Heinemann, 1996; 137–160.
13. Herrmann M, Wallesch C. Psychosocial changes and psychosocial adjustment with chronic and severe nonfluent aphasia. Aphasiology 1989;3:513–526.
14. Sarno J. The Psychological and Social Sequelae of Aphasia. In M Sarno (ed), Acquired Aphasia. San Diego: Academic, 1991; 499–519.
15. Sinyor D, Jacques P, Kaloupek D, et al. Post-stroke depression: relationship to functional impairment, coping strategies, and rehabilitation outcome. Stroke 1986;17:1102–1107.
16. Gainotti G (ed). Emotional, psychological and psychosocial problems of aphasic patients. Aphasiology 1997;11(7):[special issue].
17. Aten J, Caligiuri M, Holland A. The efficacy of functional communication therapy for chronic aphasic patients. J Speech Hear Disord 1982;47:93–96.
18. Elman RJ, Bernstein-Ellis EG. What is functional? Am J Speech Lang Pathol 1995;4:115–117.
19. Elman RJ. Memories of the "plateau": health care changes provide an opportunity to redefine aphasia treatment and discharge. Aphasiology 1998;3:227–231.
20. Avent JR. Manual of Cooperative Group Treatment for Aphasia. Boston: Butterworth–Heinemann, 1997.
21. Vickers CP. Communication Recovery Workbook. San Antonio, TX: Communication Skill Builders. (In press.)
22. Aten J, Kushner-Vogel D, Haire A, et al. Group treatment for aphasia: panel discussion. Clin Aphasiol 1981;11:141–154.
23. D'afflitti J, Weitz G. Rehabilitating the stroke patient through patient-family groups. Int J Group Psychother 1974;24:323–332.
24. Marquardt T, Tonkovich J, DeVault S. Group therapy and stroke club programs for aphasic adults. J Tenn Speech Hear Assoc 1976;20:2–20.
25. Agranowitz A, Boone D, Ruff M, et al. Group therapy as a method of retraining aphasics. Q J Speech 1954;40:170–182.
26. Aronson M, Shatin L, Cook J. Sociopsychotherapeutic approach to the treatment of aphasic patients. J Speech Hear Disord 1956;21:352–364.
27. Bloom L. A rationale for group treatment of aphasic patients. J Speech Hear Disord 1962;27:11–16.
28. Corbin M. Group speech therapy for motor aphasia and dysarthria. J Speech Hear Disord 1951;16:21–34.
29. Kearns K, Simmons N. Group therapy for aphasia: a survey of V.A. medical centers. Clin Aphasiol 1985;15:176–183.
30. Pachalska M. Group therapy for aphasia patients. Aphasiology 1991;5:541–554.
31. Bollinger R, Musson N, Holland A. A study of group communication intervention with chronically aphasic persons. Aphasiology 1993;7:301–313.
32. Wertz R, Collins M, Weiss D, et al. Veterans administration cooperative study on aphasia: a comparison of individual and group treatment. J Speech Hear Res 1981;24:580–594.
33. Elman RJ, Bernstein-Ellis EG. Effectiveness of group communication treatment for individuals with chronic aphasia [abstract]. ASHA 1996;38:52.
34. McTear M. Pragmatic disorders: a question of direction. Br J Disord Commun 1985;20:119–127.
35. Mishler E. Meaning in context: is there any other kind? Harvard Educ Rev 1979;49:1–19.
36. Prutting C. Pragmatics as social competence. J Speech Hear Disord 1982;47:123–134.
37. Prutting C. The pragmatics of language: theoretical and applied issues. S Afr J Commun Disord 1984;31:3–5.
38. Prutting C, Kirchner D. A clinical appraisal of the pragmatic aspects of language. J Speech Hear Disord 1987;52:105–119.
39. Copeland M. An assessment of natural conversation with Broca's aphasics. Aphasiology 1989;3:301–306.
40. Holland A. Observing functional communication of aphasic adults. J Speech Hear Disord 1982;47:50–56.
41. Lubinski R, Duchan J, Weitzner-Lin B. Analysis of breakdowns and repairs in aphasic adult communication. Clin Aphasiol 1980; 10:111–126.
42. Meuse S, Marquardt R. Communicative effectiveness in Broca's aphasia. J Commun Disord 1985;18:21–34.
43. Prinz P. A note on requesting strategies in adult aphasics. J Commun Disord 1980;13:65–73.
44. Smith L. Communicative activities of dysphasic adults: a survey. Br J Disord Comm 1985;20:31–44.
45. Yorkston K, Davis G. Speech act analysis of aphasic communication in individual and group settings. Clin Aphasiol 1977; 7:166–174.
46. Porch B. Porch Index of Communicative Ability. Palo Alto, CA: Consulting Psychologists Press, 1973.

47. Holland A. Communicative Abilities in Daily Living. Baltimore: University Park Press, 1980.
48. Shewan CM. Auditory Comprehension Tests for Sentences. Chicago, IL: Biolinguistic Clinical Institutes, 1979.
49. Ehrlich JS, Sipes AL. Group treatment of communication skills for head trauma patients. Cogn Rehabil 1985;3:32–37.
50. Ruff RM, Niemann H. Cognitive rehabilitation versus day treatment in head-injured adults: is there an impact on emotional and psychosocial adjustment? Brain Inj 1990;4:339–347.
51. Katz MM, Lyerly SB. Methods for measuring adjustment and social behavior in the community: I. Rationale, description, discriminative validity and scale development. Psychol Rep 1963;13:503–535.

CHAPTER TWO

Group Process, Group Dynamics, and Group Techniques with Neurogenic Communication Disorders

Susan E. Adair Ewing

It is increasingly important for speech-language pathologists to be aware of group process and group dynamics as more programs begin focusing on groups. Group process and dynamics show what occurs under the surface for our communicatively impaired clients in a treatment group. This chapter reviews the literature on groups in the fields of psychology and social work.

All of us have been group members, and some have even run groups, but many of us have had no formal training in group work. Groups unite people with similar problems to help them cope. They have evolved as a safe place for members to share their strengths and resources and receive needed support for specific problems. Groups such as Alcoholics Anonymous have a set format but no professional leader. These groups are based on the resource collaboration model [1] and are very much a part of today's culture.

In the psychotherapeutic group model, the same members meet on a regular basis in small groups facilitated by a professional leader. These groups serve more than social and support functions, because they are formed to promote growth of the individuals involved. In the neurogenic population, groups that improve functional communication also have a supportive role, as members learn about themselves in the context of disability. Groups are a powerful tool for learning and, as Luterman [2] says, the job of leader in a therapeutic group is to release the collective wisdom within. From Luterman's discussion, it is apparent that the group itself is the vehicle for learning and the relationships formed in a group promote change. Social workers Bertcher and Maple [3] affirm that groups have interdependent interaction where norms and values develop to enhance goal achievement. Change occurs as members are empowered to take responsibility for their growth. Toseland and Siporin [4] see groups as a way for individuals to form supportive relationships and, through helping others, to increase the individual's self-worth. By using role models and developing new skills, a group member explores new ways of thinking and communicating based on feedback from the leader and his or her peers.

BENEFITS OF GROUP MEMBERSHIP

Lieberman and Borman [1] interviewed people in crisis who sought out a group, in an attempt to learn what benefits they perceived from group membership. Lieberman and Borman classified the reasons that brought people to a group as *individual, cognitive,* or *communicative,* and they studied the corresponding changes that occurred after group therapy. Individual changes were defined as those that enriched connections with others; cognitive changes described learning within an intellectual framework. Communicative changes were specific styles of communicating that ensured a clearer message. Other researchers have supported Lieberman and Borman's findings and found that perceived benefits depended on whether the group was a self-help, support, treatment, or psychotherapeutic group. Individual learning includes modeling from the leader and other members'

ways of relating to others. Additional benefits include the instillation of hope, emotional support, catharsis, and universality. Hope creates a sense of optimism that life can be different. Because each group member is dealing with a similar problem, members are able to make sense of their experiences by sharing with one another.

Yalom [5] emphasizes that catharsis, although it is essential, can be overwhelming for a group unless a cohesive bond has been established among the members. He adds that catharsis alone does not help people grow and change. Yalom supports Lieberman and Borman's research that cognitive as well as individual learning is reason for seeking membership in a group. Yalom concludes that cognitive learning is a framework in which to put experiences so that long-term change can occur. In a group, cognitive learning occurs as people see how others handle problems and begin to realize how families and culture shape attitudes, beliefs, and behaviors. Group members begin to practice new behaviors and discover their personal impact on others. Communication is the third area in which changes occur as a result of group participation. This area is particularly important to clients with neurogenic disorders, who must not only relearn how to communicate but also must practice interacting with others. Self-disclosure is the communication skill that Lieberman and Borman found most beneficial. Yalom refers to it as *selective self-disclosure,* which is not just repetitious storytelling but disclosure that touches on deeper feelings. Another communication strategy is confrontation, or learning to speak clearly and directly to another. In addition, asking for and receiving feedback is a way of learning more about how one's communication affects others. Feedback, when members learn to use it effectively, enhances group cohesiveness. Other communication skills deemed important include the ability to listen empathetically, asking for more information instead of making assumptions about what others may have meant, reflecting and paraphrasing to ensure understanding, and learning to deal with interruptions. Later in the chapter, I present ways that the leader and other group members can encourage these important benefits.

GROUP PROCESS

What power does a group have to promote these changes? The answer is in the interaction of the group members; this unfolding is known as the *process.* Kemp [6] says, "group process connotes movement and change within the members of the group as well as within the group as a whole. . . . The characteristics . . . are related to the members considered individually and together. . . . Its expression is unique to each group." He adds that two or more people in a group working together on a problem have some covert or overt effect on one another. This tangible interdependence results in more than a social group because of the growth experienced as the members work together. Yalom [5] defines process as "the nature of the relationship between individuals who are interacting," as opposed to the content of the interaction. Therefore, the goal of the group is to form a cohesive bond where trust is established among the leader and members so that process can happen. Process begins as the group moves away from a question-and-answer format in which the leader is in charge and starts to use the leader only as a resource. (The role and specific functions of the leader in communication groups are discussed later in this chapter.) Yalom also discusses "here-and-now" learning in a group. He thinks of groups as a microcosm of society, because habitual ways of responding outside the group tend to be recreated within the group. When these patterns emerge, the leader or a group member can comment on the behavior. In this instance, the content of the interaction serves as the vehicle for observing and commenting on the behavior. This is referred to as a "process observation" [5], because it addresses a behavior that is defeating and often so ingrained in a person's behavior outside the group that he or she may have limited awareness of it. In a group, it is desirable to ask an individual if he or she is comfortable continuing with the observation or would prefer to return to it later. Yalom says that for "here-and-now" learning to happen, a process observation must be made about the behavior, or it is only experienced and not changed.

To exemplify process observation, let us look at an interaction in an established, cohesive group. B.C., an individual with aphasia, is interacting with W.D., an individual with right hemisphere communication deficits. B.C. is talking about starting a business but realizes he needs his wife's help to fill out orders rapidly; he is trying to find a way to become more independent despite his aphasia. W.D. immediately interrupts with suggestions, not giving B.C. a chance to finish speaking. B.C. could continue talking about starting a new job or expressing his frustration with his communication problems, but another group member made a process observation by asking B.C. if he felt that W.D. had interrupted him. B.C. said "yes!" and the discussion then moved away from content to ways to handle interruptions. The group learned that B.C. often felt that others jumped in before he finished speaking, and W.D. immediately realized that this interrupting behavior was what his family members kept commenting on. Yalom [5] would describe this as a completed loop. First, the group experienced and supported the content of the interaction, that of starting a new job and the ensuing difficulties. The interpersonal learning loop was completed by a process observation: the effect of interruptions on the aphasic individual. B.C.'s emphatic yes indicated that others finishing his sentences was most likely occurring outside the group. By staying in the "here and now," the group was able to explore the deeper meaning of the interaction and provide practice and solutions for dealing with interruptions outside the group.

GROUP PROCESS WITH THE NEUROGENIC POPULATION

In group process, it is not only the practice of communicating with disrupted communication that promotes change but also the comments about the interaction. Some modifications must be made for a population with neurogenic communication disorders. We are often dealing with people who have reduced verbal initiation, decreased communication, and short-term memory problems. Therefore, many process observations are about communicative style and how altered communication changes the group members, their relationship to their families, and their relationship with the larger community. Therefore, the leader has a different role than he or she would have in groups where the common problem is not communication loss. In groups of individuals with communication disorders, the leader must be aware of each group member's communication deficit to encourage and ensure continued interaction. For instance, a nonverbal individual may need a communication notebook, hand-held computer, or paper and pen to interact with the group. For those with an auditory comprehension difficulty, a picture or written word (or both) is needed to check understanding. In addition, group members must become increasingly aware that they may have missed information so they can begin to signal for themselves. Members' initiation skills need to be reinforced, so that the leader is not always the one who begins the exchange. The added facilitation by the leader (and eventually other group members) further reinforces "here-and-now" awareness; to improve communication, strategies need to be practiced continually in this smaller protected setting. Because brain injury makes new learning more difficult, the very nature of the sudden loss of speech and language with slow recovery makes it difficult to develop an interactive group. Initial speech therapy is usually driven by the therapist. When a speech-language pathologist is present in a group, group members expect that this is who will drive the group, just as in individual therapy. It is a new experience for group members to take responsibility for their interactions.

The advantage of group work with the neurogenic population, as psychologist Susan Wiley [7] suggests, is that after the devastation of a major illness, people feel more vulnerable and open to change. She believes that people are often willing to try new ways of being after a major illness, and many are able to be active group participants based on their increased needs. Those of us who have had the opportunity to facilitate groups know that each group is unique. Individual personalities seem to meld to form a group personality. The goal of the group leader is to form a cohesive group where members feel comfortable enough to self-disclose and where growth can occur. One important issue for the leader is deciding who fits into a particular group to ensure that a good group personality emerges. Severity level of the communication loss is one criterion used to decide membership, but it is useful to look at the energy of the prospective member as a way of deciding the makeup of the group. We all have experienced clients with limited communication who brought so much energy to their limited communication that it appeared they had more verbal ability than they really had. A group needs people with this energy to be cohesive and for process to work.

STAGES OF GROUP DEVELOPMENT

Once group members are selected and the group is ready to begin, it goes through various stages of development. Many authors have discussed stages of a good working group, and although the dynamics are similar, the stages are labeled differently. To simplify the discussion, I consider the stages of a closed group in which the same members attend throughout. With institutional pressures, it is often not possible to have a closed group. For many of us, an open group is the norm: The group continues at the same time and place, but members commit for differing amounts of time, resulting in multiple beginning and ending dates. This does have an effect on group dynamics, but usually a core group of members keeps the process going. Thus, the addition of a new member does not take the group back to the initial stages of group development. I have found that an open group actually works nicely because it gives older group members a chance to review changes and new learning as they begin to share knowledge with new members and concurrently reinforce commitment to the group.

Tuckman [8] provides easy-to-remember terminology for his stages of a good working group. He divides a group into four stages: forming, storming, norming, and performing. The first stage, forming, lasts only a few sessions, as introductions set the tone for future sessions. In the storming stage, conflicts may arise, creating a dynamic in which some members become leaders and others followers, as agreements and ways of operating within the group are set. This is when individual personalities create the group personality. In Tuckman's third stage, norming, rules are used to govern the group. Cohesiveness and cooperation as a unit are seen. In the last stage, performing, cohesiveness increases, and in an effective group, members adopt lifelong changes and ways of being.

Gazda [9] also talks about four stages: exploratory, transitional, action, and termination. In Gazda's exploratory stage, aside from the initial introductions, group parameters are established as members become aware of how the group operates. During the exploratory stage, group members start to feel safe and protected in their new surroundings. In contrast to Tuckman, Gazda believes that the role of each group member is defined during this first stage. During Gazda's transitional stage, a few of the members begin to feel comfortable and self-disclose at a deeper level, whereas others may resist this new level. The leader helps members to feel more comfortable by staying aware of the anxiety, defensiveness, and resistance of some members. In Gazda's action stage, people begin to modify their behavior, their responses to communication loss, and the nature of their long-term disability. The termination stage helps the group to work most effectively because they are aware that their time is limited. The termination stage involves summarizing and reviewing group learning and finding ways to obtain support outside the group with what they have learned in the group.

In contrast to Tuckman and Gazda, Yalom [5] delineates three group stages: inception, working, and termination. Although Yalom describes group stages, he recognizes that no single event takes a group from one stage to the next. Many groups may not develop to deeper levels of trust and disclosure, thereby limiting the progression to a subsequent stage. At times, this lack of progression may be due to the timing of the leader, but it may also be a result of the dynamics among group members. Therefore, even if considerable time has been spent choosing group members, a group may not develop the desired cohesiveness. It is interesting to note that the addition or subtraction of one member may change the dynamic of an entire group. Yalom talks about the inception stage as the time when procedural norms and structure are established. At this point, everyone is on his or her best behavior, usually waiting to see how the leader proceeds. Trust has not yet been established, so topics are introduced hesitantly and usually only touch the surface. The leader's responses are crucial at this stage, because it is tempting to move the group too quickly through the process. A group should not be pushed; it takes time for process to unfold. Yalom says that the working stage is the time when cohesiveness and conflict exist simultaneously. Contrary to what one may think, conflict in a group is a signal that group dynamics are working well, for without trust, conflict cannot emerge. Conflict helps the group address real issues and learn about compromise and resolution. Members become increasingly aware of the strengths and talents in the group and are able to use these resources. Much of the content that may have been part of the group at its inception is now addressed again at a deeper level. Yalom agrees with Gazda that the termination stage is an important part of group process. This stage needs to be handled well so that people can move on and use their changes outside the protective group environment. Separation and change are issues many of us have difficulty addressing. Clients dealing with significant adjustments because of brain injury are even more vulnerable to change. The leader needs to handle endings with understanding as the group or an individual's participation in it ends.

One client, C.B., had difficulty with termination. C.B. was a woman who had made dramatic changes in recovery of her speech and language and was showing great confidence in handling her affairs at home. When a member is planning to leave the group, I normally start the termination process at least three sessions before the final session. In this case, I had been busy and had forgotten to start this process. Because C.B. had made so many successful transitions outside the group, however, I thought that she would not be as sensitive as others to the end of her stay in the group. She was unusually quiet during her second-to-last session, but again, given my busy practice at the time, I took only fleeting notice of this change in her participation. Two days later I received a phone call from C.B. She provided a well-thought-out, carefully articulated statement of how my oversight had made her feel and how this had made her lose trust in me because she felt overlooked once again which had been a major issue for her. The group had helped her regain her sense of self, but my oversight had set her back. I decided to have her stay a few extra sessions so that she could terminate from the group properly and not lose the ground that she had gained. Her ability to deal so directly with me helped her to use her learning effectively outside the group, even with her aphasia.

ROLE OF THE LEADER IN A GROUP SETTING

The role of a leader is of utmost importance. Jourard [10] believes that the leader is a strong determiner of how the group will unfold, even though the process is the result of all the relationships formed in the group. The leader establishes the level of trust and cohesiveness that ultimately contributes to the success of the group. I view the leader as the one who sets the structure, establishes parameters, provides resources, and builds cohesiveness in the initial stages of group development. The leader must sense when it is appropriate to move the group forward, when there is enough trust to confront self-defeating patterns, and when it is appropriate to make process observations based on the group interaction. A leader should provide insight and feedback as well as help to create a supportive environment in which members feel comfortable trying new ways of communicating and bringing up problems or disappointments that result from their disability. A leader controls feedback to an extent, but he or she must always be aware of his or her own biases to make the outcome of the group interactions as fair as possible. Perhaps most important for process, groups must get away from being leader driven. At the onset, however, the leader is important in modeling acceptable behavior so that members can feel safe disclosing at a deeper level.

In their research on the desirable qualities of a leader, Cartwright and Zander [11] agree with Jourard that groups operate differently depending on the leader. They conclude that in addition to having knowledge about groups, a good leader should be flexible and acutely aware of the subtle changes occurring in a group. If the group changes, so must the leader. They suggest that in a successful group, all members share the leadership function, even though the leader exerts the most influence on the members. Kemp's [6] research supports Cartwright and Zander but adds the importance of a leader's empathy and listening with understanding. A leader is responsible for creating an atmosphere of trust with behavior that does not threaten, evaluate, or reject. Kemp feels that the leader performs an important linking function by expressing members' thoughts to add to the flow and force of interactions. The leader reflects meaning on members' statements, going beyond the content to deeper meaning. Corey and Corey [12] describe a good leader as open, undefensive, and self-aware. A good leader questions in a way that helps group members to relax; confronts; is honest, supportive, and able to block attacks from other group members; and can understand nonverbal behavior. To facilitate the group, a leader must be open to expressions of conflict and must listen, reflect, clarify, and summarize group interactions. Jourard [10] adds that it is important for a leader to have courage, presence, caring, and, above all, a sense of humor. He stresses the importance of a leader's self-knowledge of his or her therapeutic style so that he or she is free to share reactions honestly and forthrightly. His research supports these qualities as necessary for a leader to create a group in which trust can be established to promote cohesiveness and, ultimately, individual growth.

ROLE OF THE GROUP LEADER WITH THE NEUROGENIC POPULATION

The leader's role changes when he or she is dealing with individuals who have communication loss. In an ideal group, the leadership role is shared, but the speech-language pathologist may be the only member of a group who is aware of others' communication limitations. Because of these limitations, it is up to the leader to structure the group so that extra time is allowed to reiterate, clarify, and review. Often, further clarification is done by writing, drawing, or asking particular members if they understand the interactions. Eventually, individuals with special needs learn how to indicate for themselves when they need further clarification. Asking for clarification becomes a group "here-and-now" issue, and strategies to ensure understanding are practiced and reinforced for later use. To work on carryover from week to week, a leader might begin a group session by asking what was important from the previous week. This can be a problem, given short-term memory loss, but the very issue of review can help a member learn ways to manage memory. (At times, I have provided a short summary of the previous week to begin a session or kept a note for each person related to ongoing communication and social goals.) Although a silent member is common in any group, in a neurogenic group the silence may be a direct result of the communication problem. Initially, the leader may have to take on more responsibility for the silent member until such behaviors as inquiring about the reason for the silence or giving the member additional strategies for interacting can be modeled. As the leader models these behaviors, other members begin to share this role.

GROUP TREATMENT TECHNIQUES

The measure of a successful group is increased participation and interaction by all members. Bertcher [13] names specific group techniques that add to our knowledge of effective group dynamics and group participation. Many of these techniques were described earlier (see Benefits of Group Membership and Role of the Leader in a Group Setting). I expand on this review briefly to increase awareness of the dynamics of group interactions (Table 2-1).

Initially, Bertcher reviews the technique of *starting*. As a group becomes more cohesive, the routines of starting are assumed by all members, but initially this activity falls to the leader. How a group starts can determine the outcome. Therefore, the leader must know how he or she wants that

TABLE 2-1.
Bertcher's Group Techniques

Starting
Attending
Seeking and giving information
Contract negotiation
Rewarding
Responding to feelings
Focusing
Summarizing
Gatekeeping
Confrontation
Mediating
Modeling

Source: From HJ Bertcher. Group Participation Techniques for Leaders and Members (2nd ed). Thousand Oaks, CA: Sage Publications, 1994.

group to unfold in the coming weeks. For instance, my vision for a group is one where all members participate. To accomplish this, each member must have all the necessary aids to facilitate optimum communication. In addition, the group must be seated so that those with a vision impairment or hemiparesis can be comfortable and see everyone. Having a clear vision of how the group should start makes it more likely that effective process will occur.

Attending (also known as *active listening*) is basic because it demonstrates to the group that you (as leader) are aware of the message and the underlying meaning. A former client, M.A., exemplifies the dynamic of attending. In a group session, M.A. said that it was fine if his spouse chose not to attend a meeting where he was going to speak to a group for the first time since his stroke, but he said it in a voice choked with emotion. The overt message was, "I will deal with this, I have handled it before," but the underlying message was one of hurt and disappointment. To establish trust and cohesiveness, the leader must recognize the underlying message. It is up to each member to decide how much to respond, but if the real message is not acknowledged in some way, the member may lose trust in the group.

Another technique is *seeking and giving information*. Although group members may share a common problem, there are still race, age, gender, and cultural differences among members. Therefore, seeking and giving information is used to clarify an interaction based on these differences, making certain that it is clear to that member why more information is needed. In one example, group member H.T. said that he wanted a divorce. The group does not need to know everything that has led to the potential divorce, but the group does need to know how the difficult relationship affects the member's communication. Asking too many questions about the desire for a divorce is not in our area of expertise and is irrelevant to group discussion. Appropriate questioning might start with, "This is a tough issue, would you like to discuss it further?" Or one might say, "Tell me more about . . ." or "You have received a lot of feedback, would you like more?" This method of seeking and giving information is designed to help the member see the need for clarification while determining how much he or she wants to share.

Contract negotiation is usually used in the first stages of a group, because it deals with the norms and rules for membership. It allows members to feel safe in the group and understand the reason for the group's existence. Usually the leader has explained the nature of the group before the first meeting, but contract negotiation issues may appear periodically as new members are assimilated. In a group with communication disorders, it must be clear that the group exists to help with communication and to deal with psychosocial issues related to brain injury. Although premorbid personal issues cannot help but emerge in some form, it must be clear that our area of expertise is speech-language pathology.

Rewarding is closely allied with contract negotiation. It is used to increase group interaction by pointing out and reinforcing acceptable behavior. For example, if a silent member finally begins to initiate communication, this should be rewarded to reinforce the changed behavior. Another technique of Bertcher's is *responding to feelings*. This is important because if a member discloses at a deep, personal level and feels ignored, he or she may feel rejected, which would have a negative effect on the group dynamics. It is important not only to acknowledge feeling but also to make sure that the feelings expressed were interpreted correctly by the group. This relates to the technique of attending. For example, a member may say, "Am I right that you are feeling . . . ?" Milnes and Bertcher [14] talk about verbal empathetic responding. They conclude that a leader can respond to a feeling by making a mental note of the feeling to see if it reappears, acknowledging it and going on, or asking the member if further discussion is desired.

As with attending, *focusing* is most often used by the group leader. Yalom [5] calls this technique a *process observation*. It was demonstrated in the example in which B.C. discussed his problems with return to work and was interrupted by W.D. Focusing called the group's attention to the underlying message in the interaction to help reach group and personal goals. The technique of *summarizing* is closely aligned with focusing in that it reiterates important learning, but it usually occurs at the beginning and end of sessions. Summarizing is used to start the group and form a linking function with the previous week's session; at the end, it is used to reiterate responses that helped move the group forward. *Gatekeeping* is used to track member participation and important information that was shared during the session. It is similar to summarizing in that it is an observation about what has or has not happened during the session. A leader may express his or her observations about a particular experience or interaction in the session or only track it for future reference.

A technique that is often used in a cohesive group is *confrontation*, which is a way to speak clearly and directly to another member. Because confrontation is often emotionally charged, it should be used only when trust and cohesiveness have been established in the group. Conflict helps to move a group forward, and confrontation allows members to discover recurring patterns that may be impeding progress. When a member feels comfortable enough to address an emotionally charged issue in a caring and concerned way, the individual and the group can grow.

Mediating is an important component of group facilitation and is needed when there is disagreement. Mediating is a function performed by a neutral person, usually the leader. In one of my groups, there was a conflict between two members about coping with disability. The discussion was intense, and my role was to clarify each person's stance. Each person was so intent on articulating his point of view that they stopped listening to one another. As it happened, they were actually in agreement on many points, but a neutral person was needed to help sort out the various arguments that had been made to support their beliefs. Process unfolded as the members felt comfortable enough in the group to let the conflict emerge and to practice their ability to represent themselves in a group. *Modeling*, Bertcher's final group technique, has been mentioned as a perceived benefit of group participation. It is used frequently by the leader in the initial stages of group development to show members how desirable behavior should be reinforced. Modeling adds to group cohesiveness as all members begin reinforcing acceptable behavior.

Group techniques differ widely from techniques used by speech-language pathologists in individual sessions. According to Forsyth [15], this is true because of the number of individual relationships that can occur in a group. When individual change is the goal, Forsyth thinks that the optimal number of individuals in a good working group is four to nine. A cohesive group occurs when members meet regularly to work on change. Too large or small a group does not produce the optimal number of relationships to promote group interaction and growth. My experience with communication loss groups has been similar, with the best groups having 10 members at most. It takes longer for interactions to occur because of speech or language problems; therefore, having too many members in a group interferes with people having enough "air time." However, change also occurs by observation for those who are quiet during some sessions. Having too few members can take the group back to being leader driven.

PSYCHOSOCIAL ISSUES

Premorbid, unresolved personal and family issues may be more pronounced after a major disruption, such as brain injury. The ensuing losses often influence the content of group discussion. Themes that emerge frequently are changes in self-esteem and self-image. Many people begin to look at their communicative and physical changes. It is an important part of the recovery process to recognize how such changes affect relationships. Social isolation is also frequently brought up because of its prevalence in this group—because of changes in interactions with others or because of limitations on activities due to physical changes. Many people begin to feel the need for support when their familiar support systems change dramatically.

For example, they may no longer see people at work or be able to participate in the activities that they once did. New options for socialization are often topics for discussion in the group. Fears related to disability tend to be discussed frequently. These fears include appearing foolish in public when speech and movement are different or fear of having another stroke, dying, or beginning new activities. Grief is another emotion that emerges in a cohesive group. Some members are comfortable sharing their feelings of sadness, frustration, despair, anger, guilt, shame, resentment, and hopelessness. Others may be less comfortable talking about their feelings, but listening to others in the group may help their own process. Although it is not our role to "fix" these problems, our knowledge of group dynamics and group techniques should allow people the freedom to voice their innermost feelings and let both the process and healing begin. When dealing with these psychosocial issues, we need to respect our boundaries as speech-language pathologists. Many premorbid issues unrelated to the brain injury should be referred to those psychologists, social workers, or psychiatrists who are also knowledgeable about communication loss.

COMMUNICATION PRACTICE IN THE GROUP SETTING

The major impetus for creating communication loss groups is to aid recovery of communicative competence. Because interaction is at the heart of group dynamics, the group setting promotes reinforcement of communication strategies learned in individual treatment. Groups provide many opportunities to work on initiation and explanation of selected topics. Topics range from current events to life experiences and personal interests to psychosocial issues. Because group members are dealing with a group of people, they may become more aware of auditory comprehension problems that may not be so obvious in individual treatment. Group members can learn to ask for repetition or other ways of ensuring comprehension, which are strategies necessary outside the group. The group provides an opportunity for a more natural exchange of information built on the interchange among several people, not only with the leader.

CONCLUSION

Speech-language pathologists are facilitating more groups, but few have been trained in group dynamics. Groups are more than an extension of individual therapy. Group participants who have had individual treatment need to learn to become group members, just as speech-language pathologists must learn the techniques necessary to develop cohesive groups in which all members share responsibilities. Groups help individuals feel that they have more control of their lives as they gain competence in communication. Our role becomes one of observing and guiding [16] as we help the group process to happen. Group dynamics facilitate change as members gain communication skills and understand the consequences of their long-term disability.

REFERENCES

1. Lieberman MA, Borman LD. Self-Help Groups for Coping with Crisis. San Francisco: Jossey-Bass, 1979.
2. Luterman DM. Counseling the Communicatively Disordered and Their Families (2nd ed). Boston: Pro-Ed, 1991;113–133.
3. Bertcher HJ, Maple FF. Creating Groups (2nd ed). Thousand Oaks, CA: Sage Publications, 1996.
4. Toseland R, Siporin M. When to recommend group treatment: a review of the clinical and research literature. Int J Group Psychother 1989;36:171–201.
5. Yalom ID. The Theory and Practice of Group Psychotherapy (3rd ed). New York: Basic Books, 1985;135–198.
6. Kemp CG. Perspectives on the Group Process. Boston: Houghton Mifflin, 1964.
7. Wiley S. Structured treatment approach for families in crisis. Am J Phys Med 1983;62:271–285.
8. Tuckman BW. Developmental sequence in small groups. Psychol Bull 1965;63:384–399.
9. Gazda GM. Human Relations Development: A Manual for Educators (3rd ed). Boston: Allyn & Bacon, 1984.
10. Jourard SM. Disclosing Man to Himself. New York: Van Nostrand Reinhold, 1968.
11. Cartwright D, Zander A (eds). Group Dynamics: Research and Theory (3rd ed). New York: Harper & Row, 1968.
12. Corey MS, Corey G. Groups: Process and Practice. Belmont, CA: Brooks/Cole, 1992.
13. Bertcher HJ. Group Participation Techniques for Leaders and Members (2nd ed). Thousand Oaks, CA: Sage Publications, 1994.
14. Milnes J, Bertcher HJ. Verbal Empathetic Responding. Ann Arbor, MI: Campus Publications, 1975.
15. Forsyth D. Group Dynamics (2nd ed). Pacific Grove, CA: Brooks/Cole, 1990.
16. Shaffer J, Galinsky MD. Models of Group Therapy (2nd ed). Englewood Cliffs, NJ: Prentice-Hall, 1989.

CHAPTER THREE

Measuring
Outcomes
of Group Therapy

Kathryn L. Garrett

The authors of this book believe that group treatment approaches to the management of aphasia, dysarthria, and cognitive disabilities can effectively meet participants' needs and improve their communication skills. The challenge for speech-language pathologists is to substantiate their general impression that group treatment works. Insurance coverage of speech-language services in a health care setting is increasingly dependent on demonstrating important changes in clients' ability to communicate. As Golper [1] stated, "We need to face the fact that our role with neurogenic populations is being changed and could be largely curtailed without the support of convincing efficacy data."

Several studies demonstrated the overall efficacy of group therapy by administering comprehensive measures of communication performance before and after treatment [2–5]. These benchmark studies paved the way for clinicians to conduct group therapy and to replicate their findings in a variety of clinical settings. Unfortunately, it is difficult to find resources that dissect the outcomes concept into meaningful and systematic measurement procedures for the practicing clinician. Clinicians frequently conduct group treatment in addition to managing large caseloads. They seldom have time to administer lengthy tests or compare treatment approaches in a controlled, experimental manner. Groups themselves pose special measurement challenges. In the acute rehabilitation setting, for example, client participation is often inconsistent because of fragile medical status, conflict with other treatments, and discharge from the facility without warning. Even in more stable outpatient groups, activities are dynamic and complex. Relationships and communication events are constructed transactionally from moment to moment, and many variables interact. Despite these inherent challenges, it is critical for the clinician involved in day-to-day service delivery to gather meaningful change data to justify continued services and to assist in the larger effort of determining if group therapy approaches are effective.

The nature of group intervention differs from setting to setting. Group treatment offered in the acute rehabilitation or subacute setting, for example, often focuses on direct treatment of the communication disability. For example, some patients with dysarthria may practice increasing their vocal loudness when conversing with other group members. Other clinicians in the acute rehabilitation or subacute setting may encourage participants to practice communicating functional information in the medical setting, such as requesting medication or assistance. In these settings, group sessions are often relatively brief. Outpatient treatment groups, on the other hand, may focus on developing communication skills while participating in extended interactional activities. For example, in an aphasia treatment program for people with long-term aphasia, individuals might participate in a series of thematic "projects," such as teaching others how to do something over several sessions. Some outpatient groups might provide opportunities for members to converse through whichever communication modality is most effective at a given moment. Still other groups attempt to provide psychosocial support and information about the disability for members and their significant others.

This chapter addresses issues, challenges, and methodologies pertaining to the practical measurement of group therapy outcomes. It describes outcome measures relative to a framework organized by *setting* (e.g., acute or subacute rehabilitation, outpatient, and long-term care), *communication disability* (e.g., dysarthria, aphasia, cognition), and *type of outcome measure* (communication measures, such as intelligibility, interactional competence, linguistic and discourse skills, and cognitive ability; functional ability and independence level; quality of life; satisfaction; and cost-benefit ratio). Within each of these categories, quantitative outcome assessment tools and strategies are described. Some qualitative approaches to outcome assessment are also presented.

DEFINING OUTCOMES

Identifying what is important to measure in a complex behavioral milieu is the first step for the practicing clinician. *Outcome measures* are tools designed to measure changes in status attributed to a specific intervention or treatment [6]. A treatment outcome can also be conceptualized as the degree and type of change experienced after participation in a clinical treatment program [7]. Therefore, treatment outcomes are usually measured before treatment begins and after it is complete, and the difference between these pre- and post-treatment data is the ultimate outcome measure. In an ideal world, an outcome should reflect positive changes, or negative results or lack of change, that follow a period of intervention [7,8]. *Outcome measurement* can be defined as the systematic measurement and analysis of treatment outcome and subsequent use of the results to change the way care is provided [9]. Thus, outcome measurement can affect individual case management as well as service delivery for agencies or even entire clinical populations.

Treatment outcome is different from treatment efficacy data. An outcome measure simply describes what happened to an individual's status on targeted variables during a treatment protocol. *Efficacy* refers to empiric evidence that the treatment protocol actually caused the change to occur [7]. Efficacy data usually derives from administration of experimentally controlled research paradigms and is often beyond the scope of what clinicians can implement in the clinical environment. Although outcome measures do not completely represent whether group therapy was responsible for changes in participant behavior, they are the focus of this chapter because this level of measurement is the most practical for the clinician immersed in daily practice.

Identification of meaningful outcomes is influenced by the perspective of the stakeholder. *Stakeholders* are individuals who have some role in the delivery of rehabilitation services. Stakeholders can include clients, clinicians, administrators, third-party payers, family members, policy makers, employers, educators, researchers, and the general public. Blackstone [8] noted that any "top 10" list of outcome measures varies depending on which stakeholders are creating the list. For example, third-party payers, administrators, and policy makers may emphasize cost-benefit ratio. Clinicians may wish to learn if their interventions caused changes in their clients' communication disability or, from a functional perspective, whether clients have generalized functional communication skills to other settings. On the other hand, clients and family members may be interested in improving quality of life (e.g., socialization opportunities, relationships with others, feelings of self-worth, independence levels, and general sense of well-being and happiness) regardless of minute changes in behavior [10].

One of the most prominent forces in identifying the value of rehabilitation services has been the World Health Organization (WHO). Its classification of impairment, disability, and handicap [11] has become a recognized framework for conceptualizing outcomes. Frattali [12] defined and illustrated the WHO components for clients with adult neurogenic disorders as follows:

- *Impairment* is the abnormality of structure or function at the organ level. It includes paralysis, sensory loss, and deficits in language systems (aphasia), speech systems (dysarthria), swallowing, and cognition (memory loss, disorientation). Impairment is typically measured with traditional instrumental and behavioral measures.

- *Disability* means the functional consequences of impairment that cause communication problems in the context of daily life activities. It includes difficulty participating in conversation, using the telephone, and following prescriptions or recipes. Disability is typically measured with functional status measures.

- *Handicap* refers to the social consequences of an impairment or disability. It includes the loss of a job, feelings of low self-worth, role changes, and social isolation. Handicap is typically measured with quality-of-life scales, handicap inventories, and wellness measures.

A REVIEW OF SAMPLE OUTCOME MEASURES

Assessment Questions and Relevant Measures

To reconcile the points of view of various stakeholders and to identify tools for measuring behavior in group treatment, five categories of outcome measures are addressed: (1) basic communication skills; (2) functional communication ability and independence level; (3) quality of life, wellness, and adjustment; (4) customer satisfaction and needs fulfillment; and (5) cost-benefit ratio. Each category is defined and framed in terms of pertinent questions for measuring outcomes. Within each category, I identified outcome measures that the busy clinician can compile in advance, administer on-line or during brief review of videotaped sessions, summarize in short order, and compare across repeated administrations. The examples appeared to be the most adaptable to group therapy sessions. This compilation provides a representative sampling of tools in various skill areas but

does not constitute a recommendation of specific outcome measures.

Basic Communication Components

INTELLIGIBILITY AND COMPREHENSIBILITY: SAMPLE ASSESSMENT TOOLS. How understandable is the communicator? In which contexts (e.g., social, environmental, semantic, syntactic, visual only, auditory only)? Given what types of enhancements or supports?

Assessment of Intelligibility of Dysarthric Speech. The Assessment of Intelligibility of Dysarthric Speech is a tool used to measure the disability of dysarthria in a standardized manner [13]. Communicators read or repeat randomly selected words or sentences of varying length from a large selection included with the test. These samples are audiorecorded; a rater unfamiliar with the stimuli then listens to the tape and transcribes the utterances. Percentage of correctly heard utterances is calculated, yielding an overall intelligibility score for both word and sentence contexts. Because communicators are tested outside the group setting, the evaluator can only infer whether test results reflect interactive communication intelligibility.

Sentence Intelligibility Test. The Sentence Intelligibility Test [14] is an updated version of the Assessment of Intelligibility of Dysarthric Speech. It brings the sentence feature of the original test to Windows and Macintosh computer platforms. The program reports several intelligibility measurements, including percentage of intelligible words, speaking rate, and a communication efficiency ratio. Because it uses standardized sentences to elicit speech samples, group clinicians must gather this information in individual sessions. As in the preceding version, the evaluator would have to infer whether test results reflect intelligibility in face-to-face discourse. Similarly, this tool does not necessarily prove that group treatment was responsible for changes in intelligibility.

Index of Contextual Intelligibility. Hammen, Yorkston, and Dowden [15] noted that speech intelligibility of severely dysarthric speakers is influenced by external factors as well as the motor act of speaking. One such factor is the semantic context of natural communication situations. The Index of Contextual Intelligibility assesses intelligibility when semantic context is known, thereby enabling the group clinician to support his or her observations of clients with severe dysarthria in the ever-changing context of the group setting.

Conversational Rating Scale. The Conversational Rating Scale rates intelligibility, in addition to five other essential communication parameters (i.e., eye gaze, sentence formation, coherence of narrative, topic maintenance, and initiation of communication) [16]. The authors use a 1- to 9-point rating scale, with defining anchors at the 1-, 3-, 5-, 7-, and 9-point ratings. For more information, see Chapter 16 or Hartley [17]. The tool can be used to rate intelligibility and conversational competence of individual communicators in a group context.

INTERACTIONAL COMPETENCE IN CONVERSATIONAL CONTEXTS: SAMPLE ASSESSMENT TOOLS. How well does the individual initiate conversational topics? Share specific information? Communicate as efficiently as possible? Take and relinquish turns? Develop a shared focus with the communication partner? Repair communication breakdowns? How often does the individual converse?

Communication Interaction Rating Scale. The Communication Interaction Rating Scale is an informal scale (Figure 3-1), a modification of one used by Sittner and Garrett [18]. It was designed to assess a communicator's group interaction skills on a number of variables using a 7-point scale. Degree of participation, ability to convey message, use of different communication strategies, variety of communication functions, and overall communication ability are measured. Repeated administrations would allow evaluators to determine if the communicator is making progress in any of the communication variables. This measure has not been standardized.

Communicative Effectiveness Index. The Communicative Effectiveness Index (CETI) is a widely cited tool for measuring the functional communication abilities of stroke patients [19]. Its 16 scaled items measure an individual's ability to interact in four basic communication situations: conveying basic needs, communicating a health threat, life skills, and social needs. Sample items pertaining to interaction include the communicator's ability to attract attention, answer yes and no questions, get involved in group conversations, have coffee-time visits and conversations, and have a spontaneous conversation, among other skills. The article guides practitioners to create their own printed copy of the CETI. A continuous linear scale is generated for each item, and the end-points of the scale represent a continuum from "not at all able" to "as able as before the stroke." The rater marks an *X* on the line to signify the rating. According to its creators, this instrument was targeted for use by significant others of the person with the communication disabilities. The authors reported that test-retest reliability and interrater reliability were strong, although a small sample size was used. In practice, it is difficult to measure change with the tool as described, because it relies on a spatial rather than a numeric scale. Many informal modifications to this tool have been implemented by practicing clinicians, including adapting the scale to a 7-point number system so that numeric comparisons could be made more easily across repeated ratings. The impact of these modifications and the generalizability of the original results to individuals in group situations and with communication disabilities other than aphasia have not yet been systematically studied.

Conversational Skills Rating Scale. The Conversational Skills Rating Scale assesses 30 conversational skills on a 5-point scale ranging from inadequate to excellent [20]. Sample skills include speaking rate, articulation, posture, use of eye contact, facial expressiveness, speaking about partner or partner's interests, initiation of new topics, maintenance of topics, use of time speaking relative to partner, overall competence, and interactional ability. Although this scale was designed to assess communicative ability in classroom settings, Hartley [17] suggests its applicability for people with neurologic communication impairments.

Communication Performance Scale. The Communication Performance Scale [4], a modification of the Pragmatic Protocol by Prutting and Kirchner [21], assesses 13 conversational skills, including intelligibility, prosody, body posture, word selection, syntax, cohesiveness, topic, initiation of conversation, repair strategies, interruption, and listening skills, among others. Each item is rated on a 5-point scale with individually defined end-points. The reliability of this scale has not been addressed. It is reprinted in Hartley [17].

LINGUISTIC AND DISCOURSE SKILLS: SAMPLE ASSESSMENT TOOLS. Is the individual able to relay specific lexical information? Use appropriately constructed, adequately complex sentences? Organize discourse to tell a story, explain a procedure, or argue a point? Convey adequate amounts of information efficiently?

Conversational Analysis. Conversational analysis has been a mainstay technique for measuring changes in conversational parameters and linguistic skills for people with acquired communication disabilities [22,23]. Following are some of the more common indices for analysis of connected speech reported in the literature.

- Content Units: Yorkston and Beukelman [24] recommended counting content units (groupings of information that are always expressed as a unit) and content units per minute to analyze connected speech, using picture stimuli to elicit the speech sample.

- Correct Information Units: Nicholas and Brookshire [25] suggested using the Correct Information Unit (CIU) to assess the informativeness and efficiency of connected speech for adults with communication disorders. They defined CIUs as words that are intelligible in context, accurate in relation to the pictures or topic, and relevant and informative about the content of the picture or topic. Words do not have to be used in a grammatically correct manner to be included in the CIU count. They elicited CIUs using 10 types of stimuli, including single pictures, picture sequences, requests for personal information, and requests for procedural information. Nicholas and Brookshire's investigation of the reliability of the number of CIUs and related indices (e.g., percentage of CIUs, CIUs per minute) showed that interjudge scoring reliability was high, as was session-to-session stability of the measures. The index also distinguished between aphasic and non–brain-damaged speakers.

- Index of Lexical Efficiency (ILE): To obtain quantitative information about the semantic output and efficiency of individual speakers, Helm-Estabrooks and Albert [26] suggest using the ILE, which is the ratio of the total number of words in the narrative divided by the number of content units produced. Individuals who produce many words without making sense to the listener would have high ILE scores; normal adults demonstrate ILEs of approximately 3.6. Helm-Estabrooks and Albert suggested obtaining the sample via picture description. However, group clinicians may be able to adapt this

Communicator: _____   Context: _____

Rater: _____   Date: _____

Instructions: Observe the communicator in an interactive group context. Circle your rating.

1. How much did the communicator participate in the interaction?

<———>
| 1 | 2 | 3 | 4 | 5 | 6 | 7 |
| None | | | Some | | | A lot |

2. How much of the time was Communicator X able to get his or her message across?

<———>
| 1 | 2 | 3 | 4 | 5 | 6 | 7 |
| None | | | Some | | | A lot |

3. How much of the time did Communicator X take an active role in the interaction by asking questions, generating unsolicited comments, or expressing opinions?

<———>
| 1 | 2 | 3 | 4 | 5 | 6 | 7 |
| None | | | Some | | | A lot |

4. How frequently did Communicator X use different ways of communicating when trying to get his or her message across (i.e., speaking, writing, Augmentative and Alternative Communication system, etc.)?

<———>
| 1 | 2 | 3 | 4 | 5 | 6 | 7 |
| Did not use methods | | | Used some different methods | | | Used many different methods |

5. How flexible and strategic was the communicator when trying to convey messages that were not understood by listeners?

<———>
| 1 | 2 | 3 | 4 | 5 | 6 | 7 |
| Not flexible | | | Some flexibility | | | Very flexible |

6. How many communication functions (e.g., asking questions, arguing, giving advice, greeting, commenting) did the communicator use when conveying messages?

<———>
| 1 | 2 | 3 | 4 | 5 | 6 | 7 |
| None | | | Some | | | A lot |

7. How would you rate Communicator X's overall communication ability?

<———>
| 1 | 2 | 3 | 4 | 5 | 6 | 7 |
| Poor communication | | | Some communication | | | Good communication |

FIGURE 3-1. **Aphasia Group Conversational Competence Rating Scale. (Courtesy of Kathryn L. Garrett and Melinda Sittner; used with permission.)**

measure to analyze conversational samples obtained in group interactions for selected individuals.

- Index of Grammatical Support (IGS): The IGS reflects the average number of "supporting words" and grammatical morphemes in each content unit [26]. This ratio is computed by adding the total number of correct words in all content units to the number of correct endings attached to these words and then dividing by the number of content units. People who produce only content words have extremely low IGS scores.

- Conversational Turns, Initiations, Total Conversation Time, and Number of Words Spoken: Packard and Hinckley [27] expanded their conversational analysis protocol for adults with moderate and severe aphasia in an effort to assess "conversational burden," which Linebaugh et al. [28] defined as the amount of responsibility each participant has to transfer information. They included nonverbal as well as verbal productions and computed several indices: number of conversational turns per partner, percentage of total initiations per partner, percentage of total conversational time used by each partner, number of words spoken by each partner, speaking rate (words per minute) for each partner, number of CIUs, percentage of CIUs, and CIUs per minute. All measures are calculated from 10-minute conversational videotaped samples obtained from the person with aphasia and his or her spouse or caregiver on a topic of their choice. In a preliminary investigation, adults with aphasia scored significantly lower than their communication partners in rate of speech and percentage of total initiations. The people receiving the highest ratings of communication sharing obtained from the American Speech-Language-Hearing Association Functional Assessment of Communication Skills for Adults (ASHA FACS) also ranked highest on percentage of total initiations, percentage of CIUs, and CIUs per minute.

Group clinicians, particularly those who continue to treat individuals in outpatient or transition groups, may want to obtain samples of speech from typical picture stimuli, role-playing, or conversational context. They would then track some of these indices over time to determine if their clients' communication behavior changes. The reliability and validity of these measures have been investigated extensively for people with aphasia; their pertinence to people with dysarthria and cognitive-based communication impairments warrants investigation.

Informal Discourse Rating Scale. This informal tool rates nine aspects of conversational behavior, discourse structure, and lexical and syntactic ability (Figure 3-2) [29]. Parameters such as relevancy, fluency, semantic specificity, organization, and efficiency are defined. Raters then determine how much they agree or disagree that the communicator shows these communication skills. This tool was initially designed to assess the communication ability of individuals with a wide range of acquired communica-

tion disabilities in group and other discourse contexts. No empiric investigations have been conducted of its validity for assessing changes in communicative competence.

Conversational Rating Scale. See Basic Communication Skills, Conversational Rating Scale earlier for a description of this scale.

Informal Rating Criteria for Narrative Maturity. Nelson and Friedman [30] drew on the work of Applebee [31], Westby [32], and Botvin and Sutton-Smith [33] to develop a tool for categorizing the complexity of spoken narratives. Their six categories (described in Nelson [34]) include *heaps* (minimal text organization with no storyline); *sequences* (narratives with a central character, setting, and topic but few transitions and superficial time sequences); *primitive narratives* (perceptually connected characters, objects, or events with some central organization and interpretive elements); *unfocused chains* (events linked in cause-effect relationships or in true sequences but with no central theme, character, or plot); *focused chains* (sequential events with a central theme but without a strong plot or goal); and *true narratives* (integratively connected events with a central theme; well-developed plot, goals, and intentions of the characters; and a related ending). This simple system for identifying narrative types can allow clinicians to track change in the complexity of group participants' spoken narratives during group storytelling. However, no reports are available on the reliability or generalizability of the information obtained with this categoric assessment tool for adults with acquired communication disabilities.

Minimal Cognitive-Communication Competencies Checklist. The Minimal Cognitive-Communication Competencies Checklist of essential listening, language production, and verbal integration and reasoning skills was compiled by Hartley and Griffith [35] and reprinted in Hartley [17]. An observer simply indicates whether a communicator's skills are present or absent in each category. Although this tool does not incorporate a qualitative rating for each skill, it does provide an initial system for identifying skills that could be targeted in therapy. Clinicians who use this checklist as an outcome measure can report on the difference in the number of skills demonstrated by the individual before and after participation in group therapy. No validation information is presently available on this measure.

COGNITIVE ABILITY: SAMPLE ASSESSMENT TOOLS. Can the person recall essential information from the recent and remote past? Anticipate and plan for future events? Anticipate consequences of actions? Develop a sequenced plan to achieve a goal? Monitor the impact his or her behaviors have in social contexts?

Executive Function Scale. The Executive Function Scale allows raters (e.g., clinicians, the person with cognitive impairment, or communication partners) to assess an individual's executive function skills in eight areas: awareness of deficits, goal-setting, planning, self-initiation, self-inhibition, self-monitoring, ability to change set, and strategic behavior [36]. It is available in published article form. A

Communicator: _____   Context: _____

Rater: _____   Date: _____

Discourse Type: Narrative   Procedural   Conversational   Persuasive   Transactional

Directions: Circle the appropriate number as it relates to each communication parameter. A value of 7 indicates strong agreement with the statement, the midpoint indicates a moderate amount of agreement, and a value of 1 indicates the least agreement. The communicator should be encouraged to convey information via any modality.

Parameter	Agreement						
	Do not agree			Somewhat agree		Strongly agree	
Clear introduction Clearly states topic, referents, purpose at beginning of discourse	1	2	3	4	5	6	7
Relevant content Information is accurate and relevant to topic	1	2	3	4	5	6	7
Topic maintenance Maintains and relinquishes topic appropriately throughout discourse	1	2	3	4	5	6	7
Semantic specificity Uses sufficient detail and specificity of language to convey referents, events, and relationships; appropriate vocabulary	1	2	3	4	5	6	7
Fluency Uses fluent speech characterized by minimal use of audible pauses, sound and word repetitions, or sound and word revisions	1	2	3	4	5	6	7
Organization of content Ideas and information are conveyed in a logical sequence and with appropriate relational structure	1	2	3	4	5	6	7
Grammaticality Uses complex grammatical sentence structure; correctly uses syntactical structures and word order	1	2	3	4	5	6	7
Efficiency Conveys ideas and information in an understandable manner in the most appropriate amount of time; few communication breakdowns or repairs	1	2	3	4	5	6	7
Functionality and understandability Effectively conveys underlying intent via available communication modalities	1	2	3	4	5	6	7

FIGURE 3-2.   **Informal Discourse Rating Scale. (Courtesy of Kathryn L. Garrett and Jane Pimentel; used with permission.)**

continuous linear scale with three anchors (severe, moderate, and within normal limits) is provided; raters mark an X on the line to represent their judgments. Raters are also encouraged to record information about context and illustrations of specific behaviors. This scale can be administered repeatedly by marking a rating on a different copy of the scale. Evidence of progress is then obtained by visually comparing the markings from repeated administrations. Although this measure does not yield a composite score, people using the scale to assess progress can report on whether the individual has made gross categoric changes in cognitive ability (e.g., from severely impaired to moderate). This scale could easily be used in its present format to assess an individual's skills in a group setting.

Group Orientation Monitoring System. The Group Orientation Monitoring System is a tool designed to measure changes in orientation and thought organization in group settings [37]. For more information, see Chapter 15.

Galveston Orientation and Amnesia Test. The Galveston Orientation and Amnesia Test [38] is commonly used to assess post-traumatic amnesia. Gillis recommends its use as an outcome measure in orientation groups (see Chapter 15).

Scales to Evaluate Solutions to Problems. Gillis created a series of scales to use when evaluating an individual's ability to solve problems. Scale B consists of a 5-point scale ranging from very effective, with minimal consequences, to ineffective, with negative consequences. Gillis recommends encouraging the group participants to self-evaluate their solutions to problems. See Chapter 16 for more information on applying this tool.

Functional Communication Ability and Independence Level: Sample Assessment Tools

How well can the individual communicate to accomplish tasks of daily living, regardless of disability level? How effectively does the individual manage personal business and conduct community transactions? How well does he or she obtain services? How effectively does he or she function in employment settings? Social or family activities? Unfamiliar or novel activities? Is the individual able to participate in communication activities independently? In all contexts? In familiar contexts? In trained contexts? With cues or prompts? With additional supports or aids?

FUNCTIONAL ASSESSMENT OF COMMUNICATION SKILLS FOR ADULTS. The ASHA FACS consists of six basic scales and two supplemental scales that measure context-based functional communication (e.g., social communication, communication of basic needs, daily planning) on a continuum of levels of independence and qualitative levels of communication [39]. Its purpose is to provide a valid, reliable, and efficient measure of functional communication within and across communication contexts. The basic 7-point scales are supplemented with additional 5-point scales that rate the communication dimensions of adequacy, appropriateness, promptness, and communication sharing for each assessment domain. Because the ASHA FACS was designed as an observational rating scale, it lends itself well to the measurement of com-

munication skills in a group setting. Data for each domain can be averaged to yield a domain mean score; these data can be plotted on a graph to represent performance over time. One disadvantage of the scale is that its emphasis on independence of communication does not fully capture the diversity of communication strategies that some group members with severe communication disabilities use. In addition, the tool does not completely describe the subtle differences in linguistic or pragmatic competence that some group participants with mild communication disabilities can experience at the level of complex discourse.

In general, the ASHA FACS allows clinicians to obtain a relatively complete picture of the communicative competence of individual communicators in a brief period. Fisher [40] found that ASHA FACS ratings completed by aphasia group therapists and therapists conducting individual therapy did not differ, thereby indicating that this tool may be valid for both treatment contexts. For the group therapist, change data (outcomes) could be obtained by observing follow-up sessions directly or by rating from videotapes of group sessions at regular intervals.

COMMUNICATION PROBES. Lyon and colleagues investigated change in quality of life and communication in adults with aphasia after participating in a series of community or home communication activities with volunteer communication partners [41]. To obtain pre- and post-treatment data, they implemented a series of procedures that may be applicable to clinicians who must assess the functionality of communication in a group therapy setting. The researchers presented one of five possible stimulus scenarios (e.g., "You would like to go to a hardware store") to each communicator, who relayed the stimulus (via any possible modality) to a professional speech-language pathologist or to a communication partner. In this case, the experimenters rated the communicator indirectly, by assessing how well the communication partner could decipher the meaning of the message within 1-, 2-, and 3-minute time limits. Lyon et al. used an 8-point ordinal scale for scoring the communication probes. To illustrate: 8 points represents accurate, complete identification of the stimuli within the first minute; 4 points represents inaccurate, related identification of the stimuli within 3 minutes; and 1 point represents inaccurate, unrelated, and noninteractive efforts to identify the stimuli within 3 minutes. Clinicians who conduct outpatient group therapy activities could conceivably conduct similar advance assessment and follow-up probes with outpatient group members as part of standard group assessment protocol.

COMMUNICATIVE EFFECTIVENESS INDEX. For a description of the CETI, see Basic Communication Components earlier.

COMMUNICATIVE ABILITIES IN DAILY LIVING. The original version of the standardized Communicative Abilities in Daily Living 68-item test assesses language production and comprehension, cognitive skills, and some pragmatic communication features in a series of role-playing activities [42]. Although time-consuming to administer to individual communicators, the test was designed to be representative of communication behavior in naturalistic situations. This test is in the process of being revised.

Quality of Life, Wellness, and Adjustment:
Sample Assessment Tools
How well is this individual engaging in positive relationships with others? Achieving optimal participation in meaningful life activities? Achieving optimal levels of autonomy and independence? Enjoying life? Adjusting to his or her disability? Maintaining or improving physical or mental health?

PSYCHOSOCIAL WELL-BEING INDEX.   Lyon and colleagues developed an informal set of 11 interview questions that pertain to an individual's satisfaction and contentedness with life [41]. The questions are rated by the communicator on a 7-point scale, from "not very, not often, or not much" to "very much or very often." Lyon et al. noted that aphasic adults demonstrated statistically significant gains in their well-being on this questionnaire after participating in naturalistic communication activities with a volunteer.

AFFECT BALANCE SCALE.   The Affect Balance Scale is a commonly used, standardized index of well-being or happiness that consists of 10 yes-or-no questions, five that address positive affect, and five that measure negative affect [43].

OREGON HEALTH SCIENCE UNIVERSITY ACTIVITY LEVEL ASSESSMENT. The Oregon Health Science University Activity Level Assessment is a checklist (Figure 3-3) developed for the Oregon Alzheimer's Disease Center that asks a rater to code the present and past activity level of a participant in a wide variety of social activities (e.g., watching movies, following finances, playing games with a friend, attending church or synagogue, and voting) [44]. The rater chooses from a 5-point scale (0 = rarely or never, 1 = yearly, 2 = monthly, 3 = weekly, 4 = daily). Evaluators track whether an individual is participating in meaningful life activities and compares present levels of activity with those from before the onset of the communication disorder.

VISUAL ANALOGUE MOOD SCALE.   The Visual Analogue Mood Scale (VAMS) [45] for mood assessment was developed to aid in the determination of depression in neurologically impaired patients, particularly stroke patients with impaired language skills. The developers of this tool noted that the outward expression of mood may not represent internal mood states in people who exhibit neurobehavioral changes after stroke. The VAMS consists of eight simple cartoon faces that depict a neutral mood and seven faces showing various mood states (sad, afraid, angry, tired, energetic, happy, confused). The neutral face and the word "neutral" is printed at the top of a 100-mm vertical line; each mood face is printed under the vertical line near the printed word. The individual is instructed to place a mark somewhere on the vertical line to indicate his or her current mood. The final score for each scale (1–100) is the number of millimeters from the neutral pole. Validation studies [46] indicated that this scale was quickly and easily completed by people with aphasia, other neurologic impairments, or significant auditory comprehension deficits and that it revealed useful information about mood state.

CODE-MÜLLER PROTOCOLS.   The Code-Müller Protocols (CMP) [47] is a 10-item written questionnaire that asks persons with aphasia and related disorders to make some predic-

tions about their abilities to work, improve their speech, meet friends socially, function independently, cope with depression, speak to strangers, cope with frustration, and form new personal relationships, among others. Individual communicators and their significant others can categorize each parameter in terms of whether they will get much worse, a little worse, stay the same, improve a little, or improve a lot. A total CMP score is computed and thus can be easily used in comparisons over time.

PRESENT LIFE SURVEY.   Records, Tomblin, and Freese developed a 60-item survey to gather information about personal happiness, life satisfaction, and educational, occupational, family, and social status of young adults with and without language impairments [48]. The survey may have some applicability to assessing quality of life among adults with acquired communication disabilities, although the appropriateness of this tool for that purpose has not been established.

Customer Satisfaction and Needs Fulfillment:
Sample Assessment Tools
How satisfied are the client and the client's significant others with group services throughout the rehabilitation process? Did they feel that relevant goals were targeted? Is the service provider assisting the individual in a personable, professional, and respectful manner? Did the service provider assist the individual and family members in increasing their knowledge? Their comfort level? Were needs met?

AMERICAN SPEECH AND HEARING ASSOCIATION FUNCTIONAL COMMUNICATION MEASURE.   The ASHA-sponsored task force that designed the Functional Communication Measure (FCM) responded to the demands of stakeholders to gather data on customer satisfaction [49]. The FCM includes a single-page rating form that contains eight items: improvement in communication, contribution of speech-language pathology services to improvement, appropriate duration and frequency of services, experience and knowledge of the clinician, desire to pay for services even if not covered by insurance, independence level of communication, and satisfaction with services. Raters (clients, family members, or caregivers) decide how strongly they agree or disagree with each statement. The inclusion of this measure represents one of the most concerted efforts to date to gather information consistently from our most important stakeholders—consumers—and their significant others.

APHASIA NEEDS ASSESSMENT.   The field of augmentative and alternative communication has adopted the view that assessing needs is one of the most critical aspects of developing an intervention plan for people with significant communication disabilities. The Aphasia Needs Assessment tool is an example of how information from an informal interview with the communicator and his or her significant communication partners can be codified in a checklist [50]. The information can then be compared between administration intervals to determine if needs are indeed being met. This tool is not standardized; it was designed to serve as an informal supplement to the clinician who conducts a verbal interview about communication needs with communicators and their significant others.

Instructions: Using the codes below, select the number that best describes the participant's past and present level of social activity.

How frequently does/did the participant:	At present	During adult life
Listen to a radio program?	_____	_____
Follow finances or investments?	_____	_____
Listen to music?	_____	_____
Watch a favorite television program?	_____	_____
Watch a movie?	_____	_____
Spend time at a hobby?	_____	_____
Play a game with family?	_____	_____
Play a game with friends?	_____	_____
Care for a pet?	_____	_____
Have visitors?	_____	_____
Visit others at their homes?	_____	_____
Go out to eat?	_____	_____
Attend a club or group meeting?	_____	_____
Take a class?	_____	_____
Attend church or synagogue?	_____	_____
Vote?	_____	_____
Travel out of town?	_____	_____

Codes
0 = Rarely or never
1 = Yearly
2 = Monthly
3 = Weekly
4 = Daily

This instrument was developed for the Oregon Alzheimer's Disease Center with the support of National Institute on Aging grant P30 AG08017.

FIGURE 3-3.   **Oregon Health Science University Activity Level Assessment. (Courtesy of Oregon Health Science University; used with permission.)**

Cost-Benefit Ratio: Sample Assessment Tool

How many hours did the individual participate in direct therapy? In indirect or related therapy activities? For how long? How much did the treatment cost? How well was time spent within sessions? For which types of clients are the most gains being observed? For which types of treatment procedures? Was group therapy a more cost-effective method of delivering the services than other forms of therapy?

As part of its mandate to devise a comprehensive system of obtaining data for all stakeholders, the developers of the first edition of the ASHA FCM [49] also included some items related to obtaining cost-benefit information. For example, on the discharge outcome data form, data on the following items are entered for each treated patient: discharge environment, adequacy of course and duration of treatment, percentage of treatment goals met, reasons for discontinuation of treatment, and number of 15-minute units of treatment delivered in individual and group contexts. The raters are asked to assess functional communication at the time of admission; this *benefit* information can then be correlated with the *costs* of receiving services.

Compiling a Profile: Triangulation of Measures

The strength of outcome data may depend on whether the questions listed above are addressed in a comprehensive, coherent manner. Using a combination of quantitative and qualitative measures, the clinician should aim to develop a strong profile of the person with the communication disability. Rather than sampling outcomes in only one of the areas described in this section, clinicians should pool their observations and measures in several outcome domains (i.e., *triangulate* their observations) to develop a more complete picture of the client's functioning at any given time [29,51–53]. This triangulated data pool, if obtained systematically and consistently, can then be used in data comparisons with other times and settings and other individuals with communication disabilities.

OUTCOME MEASURES IN VARIOUS SETTINGS

This section illustrates specific outcome measures and approaches in three service-delivery settings (acute or subacute rehabilitation, outpatient, and transition) for persons with dysarthria, aphasia, and cognitive challenges.

General Requirements

Practitioners in complex service-delivery settings require several things of outcome measures. They need measures that are efficient, valid, believable, and important. General criteria include the following:

- Measures that are *sensitive enough* to measure change for all types and severity levels of communication disabilities
- Measures that assess *important and meaningful changes* in communication, functional ability and independence level, quality of life, satisfaction, and cost-benefit ratio
- Measures that can be administered *efficiently*, with minimal time demands or discomfort for the group participant, other information providers, or the clinician
- Measures that are *valid, reliable,* and *reasonably consistent* through repeated administrations

In addition to these general criteria, different settings have different requirements for outcome measures, as discussed in the following three sections.

Acute or Subacute Rehabilitation Setting

People with diagnoses of aphasia, dysarthria, and cognitive disabilities associated with traumatic brain injury or right cerebrovascular accident are often admitted to an acute rehabilitation unit after initial treatment at an acute care hospital. People with poor endurance or fragile health are often admitted to a subacute unit for some time (anywhere from a few days to several months) after acute hospitalization in lieu of an intensive acute rehabilitation program. In the subacute unit, patients can receive all the rehabilitation services available to people in an acute rehabilitation hospital. However, they often are not required to participate in a mandatory minimum number of therapy hours.

While participating in their rehabilitation program, individuals frequently participate in group treatment sessions. Often, group treatment sessions in the acute rehabilitation setting are relatively brief (30–45 minutes). Depending on the size of the facility and the makeup of the caseload at any given time, people with severe and mild disabilities can be grouped together. At times, people with aphasia may be grouped with patients who have dysarthria or cognitive impairments. Group treatment can focus on remediation of basic linguistic or cognitive skills. Alternatively, the group facilitator can assist participants in practicing functional communication skills that they will need when they encounter specific situations with nurses, physicians, and therapists in future long-term care or rehabilitation settings. For example, in her subacute therapy groups, Marge Graham (see Chapter 5) taught people with expressive aphasia and cognitive challenges to call for assistance or to request blankets and medicine.

Many clinicians who conduct groups in acute rehabilitation or subacute settings have minimal time to develop comprehensive, individualized treatment protocols for their group participants. They may also have little control over group referrals or client discharge times. Despite these constraints, the clinician often must report on the status of each group participant during weekly staff meetings or via written reports. Although clinicians who conduct individual treatment sessions may rely on standardized testing of linguistic skills to determine if progress is occurring, these measures shed little light on whether group participation has been beneficial.

The group clinician in the rehabilitation setting can prioritize the following features of available outcome measures:

- Efficiency of administration
- Ability to measure pragmatic or interactional communication skills
- Ability to measure emerging linguistic or cognitive skills in a general manner
- Ability to measure emerging communication needs
- Ability to measure partner wellness

Table 3-1 lists measures that could be used in a rehabilitation (subacute) setting. The emphasis in this setting is on obtaining critical information about the degree and nature of the communication disability. Functional communication is increasingly a target goal at this level of care; therefore, functional communication measures are also represented on this list. Less emphasis is placed on quality-of-life measures at this point because the individual has not yet had time to adjust to the long-term realities of an acquired communication disorder in a nonmedical setting.

TABLE 3-1.
Suggested Outcome Measures across Group Therapy Settings

Targeted Outcome Dimension	Acute or Subacute Sample Measures	Setting		
		Outpatient Settings	Transition Groups	Groups
Basic communication components				
Intelligibility	Assessment of Intelligibility of Dysarthric Speech (shortened)	X	X	—
	Sentence Intelligibility Test	X	X	—
	Index of Contextual Intelligibility	X	X	X
	Conversational Rating Scale	X	X	X
Interactional in conversation	Communication Interaction Rating Scale	X	X	X
	Communicative Effectiveness Index		X	X
	Conversational Skills Rating Scale	X	X	X
	Communication Performance Scale	X	X	X
Linguistic and discourse skills	Conversational analysis: content units, CIUs, Index of Lexical Efficiency, Index of Grammatical Support, conversational turns and initiations	—	X	—
	Informal Discourse Rating Scale	X	X	X
	Conversational Rating Scale	X	X	X
	Informal Rating Criteria for Narrative Maturity	X	X	X
	Minimal Cognitive-Communication Competencies Checklist	X	X	X
Cognitive ability	Executive Function Scale	X	X	X
	Group Orientation Monitoring System	X	X	—
	Galveston Orientation and Amnesia Test	X	X	—
	Scale to evaluate solutions to problems	X	X	X
Functional communication ability and independence level	ASHA FACS	X	X	X
	Communication probes	X	X	X
	Communicative Effectiveness Index	X	X	X
	Communicative Abilities in Daily Living	—	X	X
Quality of life, wellness, adjustment	Psychosocial Well-Being Index	—	X	X
	Affect Balance Scale	X	X	X
	Oregon Health Science University Activity Level Assessment	—	X	X
	Visual Analogue Mood Scale	X	X	X
	Code-Müller Protocols	—	X	X
	Present Life Survey	—	X	X
Customer satisfaction and needs fulfillment	ASHA Functional Communication Measure	X	X	X
	Aphasia Needs Assessment	X	X	X
Cost-benefit ratio	ASHA Functional Communication Measure	X	X	X

ASHA FACS = American Speech-Language-Hearing Association Functional Assessment of Communication Skills for Adults; CIUs = Correct Information Units.

Outpatient Treatment Groups

Outpatient treatment can be delivered in a variety of settings, including hospitals, rehabilitation clinics, university clinics, and informal locations such as libraries, churches, synagogues, and community centers. Participants in outpatient groups are often known for their motivation to continue treatment. They have begun to experience the dissonance caused by returning to their home environment with changed communicative or cognitive ability. Individuals who attend outpatient treatment groups may have renewed motivation to work on their speech or thinking skills. They may request and tackle extra homework, with the ultimate ambition of returning to normal. Other individuals may have begun to accept that they will

have to learn new ways to communicate, and they may express an interest in learning compensatory approaches to convey their ideas or remember their tasks for the day.

Although outpatient groups can be organized in many different ways (e.g., by disability type, severity, or group purpose), they are often united by the common theme of functionality. Therefore, clinicians in outpatient settings especially require outcome measures of functional change in a variety of communication parameters. In addition, stakeholders interested in efficient delivery of services need to measure cost of services and ultimate change in level of care. People with cognitive and communication disorders, as well as their communication partners and family members, may also want evidence that the communication disability is changing, and that quality of life is improving. These various needs are summarized as follows:

- Ability to measure change for all types and severity levels of communication disabilities
- Ability to measure important changes in communication ability, including these:
    The person's ability to communicate functional information outside of treatment
    Interactional skills essential for participation in meaningful social relationships, including pragmatic communication skills and the ability to use compensatory communication strategies
    Skills relevant to the individual with the communication disability and to his family, peers, or social community
    Changes in the individual's linguistic or cognitive skills
    Changes in the individual's knowledge of the disability, adjustment, and wellness
- Efficiency of administration
- Ability to obtain valid, reliable, and consistent results through repeated administrations

Clinicians who see clients for the longer term in outpatient group settings are in particular need of a sample of tests that covers most of the categories described earlier: status of basic communication skills, functional communication, quality of life, and satisfaction. If possible, clinicians need to compile a selected range of tools and readminister them to obtain indices of change and justification for continued treatment. Cost-benefit information is also typically required at this stage. See Table 3-1 for sample measures.

Transition and Support Groups

People who participate in transition or support groups, particularly individuals who are recovering from and adapting to the sequelae of head injuries, typically encounter many situations that challenge their independence, problem-solving ability, and communication skills. People in these groups may no longer be funded through the traditional health care system. Frequently, support groups continue to function without formal funding because of the hard work and good graces of the participants, family members, and clinicians. Sessions often are held during evening hours in unusual locations. Other agencies may be involved, such as vocational rehabilitation. Sometimes psychologists or social workers assist in facilitation of support and transition groups. Psychosocial issues and life needs become paramount. Requirements are similar to those of outpatient treatment groups listed above.

See Table 3-1 for sample measures that meet these criteria.

CONCLUSION

It is critical for the developers of model-driven group treatment programs to incorporate strategies and meth-ods for documenting change in their participants. Group therapy sessions are rich sources of information about the dynamics of communication among individuals with communication disabilities. As treatment vehicles, they are testing grounds for a wide variety of intervention strategies, such as use of contextual information, verbal scaffolding strategies, topical suggestions, peer modeling, counseling and information provision, psychosocial continuity and support, and other independent variables. The effectiveness, impact, and efficiency of this method of service delivery must be proven. This chapter presents a preliminary framework for assessment of group treatment outcomes using a combination of old and new tools. Clinicians and researchers are encouraged to form partnerships and continue the quest to develop and standardize appropriate and useful outcome measurement tools, as well as to report on the changes in communication status for communicators after participation in group therapy programs.

Acknowledgments
Special thanks to Marge Graham for her assistance in conceptualizing and generating ideas for this chapter.

REFERENCES

1. Golper L. Message from the coordinator. Neurophysiology and Neurogenic Speech and Language Disorders Special Interest Division Newsletter 1994;4:1.
2. Bollinger R, Musson N, Holland A. A study of group communication intervention with chronically aphasic persons. Aphasiology 1993;7:301–313.
3. Elman RJ, Bernstein-Ellis E. Effectiveness of group communication treatment for individuals with chronic aphasia. A presentation at the Seventh International Aphasia Rehabilitation Conference, Boston, 1996.
4. Ehrlich J, Sipes A. Group treatment of communication skills for head trauma patients. Cogn Rehabil 1985;3:32–37.
5. Wertz R, Collins M, Weiss D, et al. Veterans Administration cooperative study on aphasia: a comparison of individual and group treatment. J Speech Hear Res 1981;24:580–594.
6. Frattali CM, Cornett B. Improving Quality in the Context of Managed Care. Managing Managed Care. Rockville, MD: American Speech-Language and Hearing Association, 1994;33–42.
7. Campbell TF. Functional treatment outcomes for young children with communication disorders. Presented at the Academy of Neurogenic Communication Disorders and Sciences, Orlando, FL, 1995.
8. Blackstone S. AAC outcomes: definition and the WHO. Augmentative Communication News 1994;8:1–6.
9. Hicks DM, Benjamin K, Aram DW, et al. Using outcome measures for assessing treatment effectiveness. Short course at the American Speech-Language and Hearing Annual Conference, New Orleans, LA, 1994.
10. Lyon JG. Communication use and participation in life for adults with aphasia in natural settings: the scope of the problem. Am J Speech Lang Pathol 1992;1:7–14.
11. World Health Organization. International Classification of Impairments, Disabilities, and Handicaps: A Manual for Classification Relating to the Consequences of Disease. Geneva, Switzerland: World Health Organization, 1980.
12. Frattali CM. Measuring disability. Neurophysiology and Neurogenic Speech and Language Disorders Special Interest Division Newsletter 1996;6:7.
13. Yorkston KM, Beukelman DR. Assessment of the Intelligibility of Dysarthric Speech. Tigard, OR: CC Publications, 1981.

14. Yorkston KM, Beukelman DR, Tice R. Sentence Intelligibility Test [Windows software]. Tice Technology Services (Lincoln, NE), 1997.

15. Hammen V, Yorkston KM, Dowden P. Index of Contextual Intelligibility. Dysarthria and Apraxia of Speech: Perspectives on Management. Baltimore: Paul H. Brookes, 1991;43–53.

16. Erlich J, Barry P. Rating communication behaviours in the head-injured adult. Brain Inj 1989;3:193–198.

17. Hartley LL. Cognitive-Communicative Abilities following Brain Injury. San Diego, CA: Singular Publishing Group, 1995;96–99, 262–263.

18. Sittner M, Garrett KL. Perceptions of the interactional competence of persons with aphasia. Presented at the American Speech-Language and Hearing Association Annual Convention, Seattle, WA, 1996.

19. Lomas J, Pickard L, Bester S, et al. The Communication Effectiveness Index: development and psychometric evaluation of a functional communication measure for adult aphasia. J Speech Hear Disord 1989;54:113–124.

20. Spitzberg BH, Hurt HT. The measurement of interpersonal skills in instructional contexts. Commun Educ 1987;36:28–45.

21 Prutting C, Kirchner D. A clinical appraisal of the pragmatic aspects of language. J Speech Hear Disord 1987;52:105–119.

22. Boles L. Conversation analysis as a dependent measure in communication therapy with four individuals with aphasia. Asia Pacific J Speech Lang Hear 1997;2:43–61.

23. Brookshire RH, Nicholas LE. Speech sample size and test-retest stability of connected speech measures for adults with aphasia. J Speech Hear Res 1994;37:399–407.

24. Yorkston KM, Beukelman DR. An analysis of connected speech samples of aphasic and normal speakers. J Speech Hear Disord 1980;45:27–36.

25. Nicholas LE, Brookshire RH. A system for quantifying the informativeness and efficiency of the connected speech of adults with aphasia. J Speech Hear Res 1993;36:338–350.

26. Helm-Estabrooks N, Albert ML. Manual of Aphasia Therapy. Austin, TX: Pro-Ed, 1991;168.

27. Packard ME, Hinckley JJ. Measuring conversational burden in adults with moderate and severe aphasia. Presented at the American Speech-Language and Hearing Annual Convention, Boston, 1997.

28. Linebaugh CW, Kryzer KM, Oden SE, Myers PS. Reapportionment of Communicative Burden in Aphasia: A Study of Narrative Interactions. In R Brookshire (ed), Clinical Aphasiology Conference Proceedings. Minneapolis, MN: BRK Publishers, 1982;4–9.

29. Garrett KL, Pimentel J. A triangulated model of outcome assessment in aphasia. Presented at the American Speech-Language and Hearing Association Annual Convention, Orlando, FL, 1995.

30. Nelson NW, Friedman KK. Development of the Concept of Story in Narratives Written by Older Children [unpublished paper]. Kalamazoo, MI: Western Michigan University, 1988.

31. Applebee AN. The Child's Concept of Story. Chicago: University of Chicago Press, 1978.

32. Westby CE. Development of Narrative Language Abilities. In GP Wallach, KG Butler (eds), Language Learning Disabilities in School-Age Children. Baltimore: Williams & Wilkins, 1984;103–127.

33. Botvin GJ, Sutton-Smith B. The development of structural complexity in children's fantasy narratives. Dev Psychol 1977;13: 377–388.

34. Nelson NW. Childhood Language Disorders in Context: Infancy through Adolescence. New York: Macmillan, 1993;429–431.

35. Hartley LL, Griffith A. A functional approach to the cognitive-communicative deficits of closed head injured clients. Texas J Audiol Speech Pathol 1988;14:42.

36. Pollens RD, McBratnie BP, Burton PL. Beyond cognition: executive functions in closed head injury. Cogn Rehabil 1988;6:26–32.

37. Corrigan JD, Arnett JA, Houck LJ, Jackson RD. Reality orientation for brain injured patients: group treatment and monitoring of recovery. Arch Phys Med Rehabil 1985;66:626–630.

38. Levin HS, O'Donnell VM, Grossman RG. The Galveston Orientation and Amnesia Test: a practical scale to assess cognition after head injury. J Nerv Ment Dis 1979;167:675–684.

39. Frattali CM, Thompson CK, Holland AL, et al. Functional Assessment of Communication Skills for Adults. Rockville, MD: American Speech-Language-Hearing Association, 1995.

40. Fisher LF. Ratings of functional communication in aphasic individuals by individual therapists, group therapists, and familiar conversational partners. Presented at the American Speech-Language-Hearing Association Annual Conference, Seattle, 1996.

41. Lyon JG, Cariski D, Keisler L, et al. Communication partners: enhancing participation in life and communication for adults with aphasia in natural settings. Aphasiology 1997;11:693–708.

42. Holland AL. Communicative Abilities in Daily Living. Baltimore: University Park Press, 1980.

43. Bradburn NM. The Structure of Psychological Well-Being. Chicago, IL: Aldine, 1969.

44. Fox LE, Fried-Oken M. Interactive group treatment for aphasia: an AAC alternative. Presented at the Seventh Biennial Conference of the International Society for Augmentative and Alternative Communication, Vancouver, BC, Canada, 1996.

45. Stern RA, Arruda JE, Hooper CR, et al. Visual analogue mood scales to measure internal mood state in neurologically impaired patients: description and initial validity evidence. Aphasiology 1997;11:59–71.

46. Stern RA, Rosenbaum J, White RF, Morey CE. Clinical validation of a visual analogue dysphoria scale for neurologic patients [abstract]. J Clin Exp Neuropsychol 1991;13:106.

47. Code C, Müller M. The Code-Müller Protocols: Assessing Perception of Psychosocial Adjustment to Aphasia and Related Disorders. London: Whorr, 1992.

48. Records NL, Tomblin JB, Freese PR. The quality of life of young adults with histories of specific language impairment. Am J Speech Lang Pathol 1992;1:44–53.

49. Kreb RA (ed.) A Practical Guide to Applying Treatment Outcomes and Efficacy Resources. Rockville, MD: American Speech-Language-Hearing Association, 1996.

50. Garrett KL, Beukelman DR. Adults with Severe Aphasia. In DR Beukelman, P Mirenda (eds), Augmentative Communication: Management of Severe Communication Disorders in Children and Adults. Baltimore: Paul H. Brookes, 1998;465–499.

51. Gliner JA. Reviewing qualitative research: proposed criteria for fairness and rigor. Occup Therapy J Res 1994;14:78–90.

52. Wilson HS, Hutchinson SA. Triangulation of qualitative methods: Heideggerian hermeneutics and grounded theory. Qualitative Health Research 1991;1:263–276.

53. Elman RJ. Multimethod research: a search for understanding. Clin Aphasiol 1995;23:77–81.

CHAPTER FOUR

Group Treatment Reimbursement Issues

Cynthia Busch

The bottom line for any speech-language pathology services, whether individual or group format, is whether the services are being paid for. The usual third-party payers are Medicare, the federal health insurance program for elderly and disabled people; Medicaid, the state-controlled health program for people in financial need; and private insurance companies or managed care organizations (MCOs). All these payer organizations cover individual and group treatment of neurogenic communication disorders in some circumstances, but they delineate very specific requirements for coverage.

MEDICARE

The following excerpt is the only guideline that specifically applies to coverage of group treatment for Medicare patients [1]:

> Group Treatment: Generally, group therapy treatment and attendance at social or support groups, such as stroke clubs or lost cord clubs, are not payable. Ensure that the "reasonable and necessary" requirements are met.

This statement clearly indicates that group treatment is reimbursable if the basic requirements for coverage of any speech-language pathology services are fulfilled. All Medicare coverage decisions are based on general guidelines, which include the following major principles:

1. General: Services must be necessary to diagnosis and treatment of communication disabilities and swallowing disorders and must be based on a specific written plan that must be signed by the patient's physician every 30 days.
2. The following conditions must be met for services to be considered reasonable and necessary:
   - Services must meet accepted standards of practice for specific and effective treatment.
   - Services must be of a complexity that requires a qualified speech-language pathologist.
   - There must be expectation of significant improvement in a reasonable period, or the services must be necessary to establish a safe and effective maintenance program.
   - The amount, frequency, and duration of the services must be within accepted standards of practice [2].

For both the provider of speech-language pathology services and the reviewer of service claims, the application of these general guidelines depends on the interpretation of certain words, such as *accepted* and *significant*. The Health Care Finance Administration (HCFA), the administrative organization for Medicare, publishes manuals for providers (e.g., the Medicare Hospital Manual) that give more specific help in interpreting policy and coverage guidelines for Medicare services.

Medicare coverage of group treatment is possible as long as all the general guidelines and "reasonable and necessary" requirements are met. It is especially important that group treatment activities be based on a carefully individualized plan of treatment designed as a result of diagnostic findings for each patient. Although specific billing procedures are not stated, it is presumed that group treatment for Medicare patients is billed at a lower rate than individual treatment. Billing procedures should clearly reflect that difference.

If all the general requirements and the "reasonable and necessary" conditions have been met, treatment groups consisting of people with motor speech disorders, aphasia, right hemisphere dysfunction, or traumatic brain injury (TBI) could be considered coverable service under Medicare guidelines. My recent review experience as the speech-language pathology Medicare consultant in Minnesota,* however, suggests that current practice patterns do not often include group treatment for Medicare patients with any of these diagnoses.

Based on my experience as a Medicare reviewer since 1981, I've compiled the following general recommendations that may help you choose appropriate treatment candidates (for group or individual services). These suggestions also may help you provide more complete documentation to support the reasonableness and necessity of the services you provide.

Careful documentation of medical history and of assessment findings is crucial. Important medical history includes the following information: pertinent medical and communication diagnoses, date of onset or date of recent change in communicative function, a description of the patient's level of communicative function before this onset or change in abilities, and the history of evaluations or treatment efforts from any previous speech-language pathology provider.

Some Medicare certification and recertification forms (HCFA Medicare Outpatient Rehabilitation Service claim forms 700 and 701) specifically require all of this medical information. Whether or not you use these HCFA forms, inclusion of this information allows efficient processing of claims at all levels of review. These federal forms for submission of rehabilitation claims have not been mandated; however, providers who submit their claims electronically are required to use them and must obtain the appropriate software from their Medicare intermediary to do so.

According to Medicare guidelines, documentation of the initial assessment must include objective baseline data from standardized or more informal measurement tools, interpretation of test results, and a narrative description of clinical findings. The communicatively impaired individual's status as a treatment candidate depends on the medical history, baseline assessment data, and whether the

---

*As of August 1998, the following states have Medicare intermediaries who employ speech-language pathologists as reviewers: California, Delaware, Florida, Georgia, Illinois, Iowa, Kansas, Michigan, Minnesota, Nebraska, New York, North Carolina, Ohio, Oklahoma, Pennsylvania, Rhode Island, Utah, Virginia, Washington, and Wisconsin. In addition, some speech-language pathology reviewers work for Medicare intermediaries who have multistate contracts.

overall findings indicate expected significant rehabilitation potential.

If the onset of the communication diagnosis is recent, at least a brief trial treatment effort is generally considered appropriate. If the onset of the communication disorder is not recent, there must be adequate justification of why services are being undertaken at that point. Acceptable rationales for initiation of treatment with a patient who has a chronic communication disorder include documentation of a recent change in medical, communicative, or cognitive function. Other factors that should be considered in determining appropriateness of treatment (for either group or individual format) include the patient's overall medical condition, the severity of the disorder, and documentation of the patient's response to previous treatment efforts.

Justification for use of the group treatment format should be explicit. Rationales for this approach might include a need for cost saving or the patient's need to practice carryover strategies learned in individual treatment into more functional communication situations with other people.

Indeed, the fact that group treatment is a sensible approach to working on functional communication among multiple partners should be explained in the supporting documentation. Medicare coverage guidelines for speech-language pathology services emphasize the need to focus on functional goals [2]:

> Functional goal: must be written by the speech-language pathologist to reflect the level of communicative independence the patient is expected to achieve outside of the therapeutic environment. Functional goals reflect the final level the patient is expected to achieve, are realistic, and have a positive effect on the quality of the patient's everyday functions.

Documentation of significant gains in functional communication skills is key to coverage of any speech-language pathology service for Medicare patients. If the patient makes such gains, and they are well documented, services in individual or group format should be coverable under Medicare guidelines.

MEDICAID

Medicaid, the federally funded health care program for persons with financial need, has state-specific criteria for coverage. In Minnesota, the Medicaid program falls under the general name of Minnesota Health Care Program (MHCP).

Under MHCP guidelines for speech-language pathology rehabilitation services, group speech-language services are covered if information is provided about the number of group members and specific documentation is included in each client's record. General guidelines that apply to all speech-language services must also be fulfilled. These guidelines require a written medical referral and a plan of care. The plan of care must include medical diagnosis, description of the patient's functional status, objec-

tives of the treatment, and documentation of progress. Also, the recipient's functional status must be expected to progress toward the stated objectives within 60 days [3].

Medicaid programs generally have significant limitations in the number of hours of service covered in a calendar year. These limitations vary greatly from state to state. For instance, in Minnesota, both individual and group speech-language services have a basic threshold limit of 50 hours (200 fifteen-minute units) on rehabilitative services for each calendar year. If a recipient needs services that exceed the 50-hour-per-year limit, the provider must make a written request for authorization before any further services are provided.

Two well-established speech-language pathology group treatment programs in Minnesota are reimbursed by the MHCP when the recipients meet eligibility requirements. Both are multidisciplinary outpatient programs that are approximately 6 months in duration and are designed to promote community re-entry for the enrolled participants.

Because most of the participants have had TBI (some have had anoxic cerebral vascular events or aneurysms), the speech-language pathology programs are focused on improving the cognitive-based language skills that are necessary to function with increased independence. Due to the cognitive nature of the treatment approach, in at least one of these programs, MHCP reviewers have required speech-language pathology services to be billed under a MHCP mental health code rather than a speech-language pathology code. This difficulty has developed because cognition falls outside of the speech, language, and hearing functions delineated in the MHCP guidelines for coverage.

MHCP reviewers have placed many other requirements on the community re-entry program administrators so that these administrators must gain prior authorization for participants. The reviewers have required specific information about program philosophy and goals, program design, the role of each discipline in the program (e.g., speech-language pathology, neuropsychology, counseling, occupational therapy, recreation therapy), billing procedures, and pertinent supporting outcome data from previous clients. Specific information that supports the need for the intensive nature of the program must be supplied.

As with Medicare guidelines, MHCP guidelines stress the need for the provider to address the recipient's functional communication status. The MHCP Provider Manual defines *restorative therapy* as follows [3]:

> A health service that is specified in the recipient's plan of care by a physician and that is designed to restore the recipient's functional status to a level consistent with the recipient's physical or mental limitations. . . . [Functional status is] the ability of the person to carry out the tasks associated with daily living.

From the reviewer's point of view, whether the speech-language pathology services are being submitted to Medicare or to one of the Medicaid programs, documentation of progress must be based on long-term functional communication goals.

Documentation of group treatment must provide clear evidence that the speech-language pathology service is making a difference in the person's ability to communicate functionally in everyday situations with other people, not just with the clinician in the treatment room.

OTHER HEALTH CARE PAYERS

Other health care payers (e.g., MCOs, fee-for-service insurance companies, and workers' compensation programs) may cover speech-language pathology services, but only if those services are indicated in the contracts developed with the employer or the client. Limits usually are placed on the number of visits or number of hours payable within a calendar year, particularly with MCOs [4]. Often, coverage can be extended by following preauthorization procedures and providing specific documentation. Coverage of speech-language services depends in part on diagnosis; adult patients with neurogenic diagnoses of stroke, TBI, or neurologic disease are likely to have covered services. Generally, both individual and group formats are acceptable as long as the service is included in the contract and other coverage guidelines are met.

In Minnesota, two outpatient community re-entry programs for groups of adults with neurogenic communication disorders are being paid for by these other payer sources (MCOs, fee-for-service insurers, and workers' compensation). The most frequent medical diagnoses of the participants in these programs are TBI, anoxic event, and aneurysm. Discussion with reviewers from several MCOs provided insight into how financial support has been achieved for such group treatment programs.

If the participant's insurance or contract includes speech and language service, the guidelines for coverage are very specific, elaborate, and subject to stringent time limits. Requirements for preauthorization (and reauthorization) may include extensive program description, specific billing procedures (lower units or per-unit cost for group treatment), submission of all participant evaluations (progress reports, re-evaluations, and discharge summaries), and specific support for the intensive nature of the program. In addition, weekly notes from each group are expected to emphasize measurable improvements in functional communication; and summaries of admission and discharge functional outcome data from previous participants in the program should be provided [4].

Claim reviewers and group treatment program administrators both mentioned an ongoing significant challenge in the authorization process. Predictably, community re-entry programs have a major focus on treatment of cognitive processes. Because the cognitive label does not fit easily into the descriptions of usual speech, language, and hearing activities, there has been difficulty obtaining agreement that cognitive services would be covered when provided by a speech-language pathologist. This difficulty appears to be a continuing one and has not yet been completely resolved.

The program administrators' education of reviewers has been and will continue to be necessary to explain the speech-language pathologist's pivotal role in treatment of the cognitive-based language skills that are basic to functional communication. In my discussions with several MCO reviewers, it became clear that those who had established relationships with speech-language pathologists from these group treatment programs were supportive (even enthusiastic) about the programs' success. In my discussions with the speech-language pathologists, it was also clear that establishing such a relationship was a long and difficult process that required them to do their homework and communicate effectively.

SUMMARY

Group treatment for people with neurogenic communication disorders is reimbursable under most third-party payment sources. Health care sources that cover individual speech-language services also cover group treatment as long as all basic requirements for coverage are met. For instance, under Medicare guidelines, group treatment is considered a covered service as long as all "reasonable and necessary" requirements are fulfilled and a fully individualized plan of treatment is implemented.

A noteworthy trend in reimbursement is the increasing number of MCOs that manage cases for people receiving speech-language pathology services in either individual or group format. If speech-language pathology is a covered service in a client's contract, generally a minimum number of visits or hours are payable in a calendar year. These services usually can be extended by following extensive preauthorization procedures.

MCOs and other payers, such as Medicaid, increasingly require weekly or monthly documentation that emphasizes measurable improvement in functional communication. Associated with this trend is a growing demand to provide admission and discharge functional outcome data for the speech-language services being used. Clearly, the clinician is challenged to fulfill demands for more and different types of high-quality documentation [4]. Therefore, although appropriate group treatment is likely to be reimbursable, the price may be high in terms of the providing clinician's work requirements.

REFERENCES

1. Medicare Intermediary Manual (Transmittal No. 1424). Washington, DC: Department of Health and Human Services, Health Care Finance Administration, 1991;Section 3905.10.C.
2. Medicare Part A Intermediary Manual (Transmittal No. 942). Washington, DC: Department of Health and Human Services, Health Care Finance Administration, 1989;Section 3101.10A.
3. Minnesota Health Care Provider Manual (1995 ed). Minneapolis, MN: Minnesota Department of Human Services, Rehabilitation Services, 1995;Section 6403.04.
4. American Speech-Language-Hearing Association Curriculum Guide to Managed Care. Rockville, MD: American Speech-Language-Hearing Association, 1996;31–40.

SECTION II

Aphasia

Part One: Speech-Language Pathologist–Facilitated Groups

CHAPTER FIVE

Aphasia Group Therapy in a Subacute Setting: Using the American Speech-Language-Hearing Association Functional Assessment of Communication Skills

Marjorie A. Graham

PHILOSOPHY OF PROGRAM

Group therapy for any type of disability offers a special challenge to the clinician. In-patient groups are particularly difficult to plan and execute. Shortened lengths of stay may create havoc with scheduling and development of cohort groups. Third-party reimbursement of group therapy is often limited to the acute phase. The program described in this chapter is a composite of a number of groups that I have conducted in subacute and skilled nursing facilities (SNFs). These groups are developed in SNFs for clients who have demonstrated potential for functional communication gains through rehabilitation services. In the subacute and SNF settings, individuals with aphasia may be in an acute stage of recovery and may remain in the setting for a sufficient number of weeks to allow for successful group interaction.

The subacute level of care is a relatively new and growing classification. The definition of *subacute* constantly changes as hospitals and traditional SNFs redefine their bed configuration to provide services to stroke patients admitted under Medicare Part A. As demand changes, providers designate freestanding or dedicated floors or wings in hospitals and nursing homes to this classification. One definition of subacute care is "intensive nursing services to patients whose conditions have stabilized beyond the need for acute care, but who require services more intensive and technologically advanced than that which the traditional nursing facility typically provides" [1]. To date, the Joint Commission on Accreditation of Healthcare Organizations is the only credentialing body to set guidelines for delivery of subacute services. As a rule, patients are admitted to a subacute rather than an acute rehabilitation unit because they cannot tolerate more than 3 hours of therapy daily. Although some stroke patients are similar to those in the hospital acute rehabilitation unit, many patients in a subacute unit do not progress rapidly to home discharge, or they require long-term care placement at the end of rehabilitation.

Stroke is one of the diagnostic categories appropriate for the subacute setting. Facilities vary greatly in the number of patients with strokes they can handle. Often, traditional long-term care facilities do not provide comprehensive rehabilitation services but will admit an occasional individual with rehabilitation potential. Other SNFs provide a full range of therapies. Depending on facility marketing skills, negotiation of managed care contracts, and regional practices, the individual with aphasia may be managed as a stroke patient in an acute rehabilitation hospital or a subacute facility. As providers negotiate with health maintenance organizations, the subacute setting may attract payers because it costs less than hospital-based programs. No matter what the political climate, clients with rehabilitation potential may be found in a variety of SNFs that are deemed subacute or long-term care.

Comprehensive communication services in an SNF are the exception. The group therapy program described in this chapter began as a 40-bed brain injury program attached to a long-term care facility. This evolved into a subacute unit. In this facility's era of providing treatment for traumatic brain injury (TBI), group therapy was an intrinsic part of the patient's daily schedule. As the facility phased out the TBI program and dedicated the beds to subacute care, the speech-language pathology department continued to conduct group therapy five times weekly to complement individual therapy. The functional nature of the groups and the emotional support they provided were a source of referrals and a focus of interest from families, staff, and administrators.

With precious few funded visits authorized by third-party payers, why would speech-language pathologists choose group over individual sessions? Group therapy has several advantages over individual therapy:

• Patient mentoring
• Peer modeling and pressuring
• Opportunity for family observation and education
• Error awareness and correction
• Contextual cues
• Group problem solving
• Reduced pressure and confrontation

Members of groups provide one another with true empathy and knowledge. During the time that I led groups, I discovered that one or two members tended to surface as the compassionate host. These mentors modeled *total communication* and provided evidence that aphasia does not necessarily ruin one's sense of humor. Mentors are needed most with severely affected individuals who require alternative modes of communication. In the individual session, clients may resist acceptance of nonlinguistic methods to convey information. Families and staff confront us with the demand, "You are the *speech* pathologist; work on his *speech!*" In groups, individuals with fluent aphasia become willing to collaborate, and they model pointing, gesturing, or drawing.

Observation of therapy by a loved one is needed to bridge the gap between therapy and the outside world, especially when training the primary caregiver. However, one-to-one sessions often lead to tears, as the client or spouse considers each error a disappointment. Family members are invited to observe groups to witness their loved ones abandon aphasia and join cohorts in an activity. In the aphasia group, this *victim* of aphasia is a member of a compassionate social group, follows recognized group rules, and succeeds in conveying information to others.

Conversation, role-playing, or structured scripts are organized around topics guaranteed to evoke a rich variety of unexpected connections. The salient information can be organized by quick-thinking clinicians to identify the value of each response. We used a grease board to organize group responses. Members are encouraged to vote on the most effective details or responses.

One-to-one sessions require that both the speech-language pathologist and the individual with aphasia remain constantly aware. There may be little opportunity for the client to relax attention skills without careful planning by the clinician to control manner of delivery and number of stimuli. During group treatment, the atten-

TABLE 5-1.
Functional End-Points for Aphasia Treatment

- Signals and gets help in an emergency (e.g., can call 911 and succeed in getting somebody to come)
- Discloses feelings (e.g., can make likes and dislikes known)
- Demonstrates retained competencies that are masked by aphasia (e.g., with maximum support from others, can get enough across to make it clear that he or she is competent to keep power of attorney, sign release forms, and participate, to whatever limited degree, in conversational interchange)
- Expresses needs (e.g., can communicate that he or she is hungry, tired, wants some time alone)
- Writes own name (e.g., can sign release forms, checks)
- Follows current events of interest (e.g., can read newspaper headlines or follow events on television)
- Derives some pleasure from activities that were pleasurable before aphasia (e.g., can demonstrate pleasure in grandchildren)
- Participates in social interactions (e.g., with maximum support from others, can demonstrate a degree of enjoyment in social interaction commensurate with pretraumatic level)
- Asserts autonomy and independence, if not of action, at least of thought and opinion (e.g., can signal disagreement, differences of opinion, take an unpopular stand)
- Forgets about being aphasic for at least limited periods (e.g., can assume a societal role in circumstances in which aphasia can be minimized, such as attending church or movies with some sign of benefit, participating in limited ways in conversation)
- Assumes some responsibility (e.g., can be expected to put out the cat or feed the fish)
- Follows simple instructions (e.g., can be expected to take own medications correctly)
- Self-monitors (e.g., knows when he or she has communicated or failed to communicate)
- Verifies understanding
- Corrects misinformation

Source: Adapted from A Holland. Functional end points. Presented at the Conference on Aphasia Treatment: Clinical Effectiveness in the New Health Care Environment, Cortland, NY, 1996. Used with permission.

tional burden is shared with other members, and clients may heighten or decrease their vigilance to stimuli. In the aphasia group, nonconfrontational tasks may be more easily performed as the clinician throws out a topic to the group. A person who responds poorly to direct imitative or responsive tasks may surprise staff, other members, and himself or herself when he or she is not the direct target of the stimulus.

Clients become wonderfully expert at error detection in others. In group therapy, they learn to detect accuracy and approximation; quietly predict the difficulty level of the stimuli; offer answers, clues, or corrections; or show utter amazement when severely affected people respond appropriately. Group members also are known to display a wide range of indirect and direct cueing strategies.

The framework of our aphasia groups is greatly influenced by the following:

- Functional communication therapy (FCT)
- Functional end-points in aphasia treatment
- American Speech-Language-Hearing Association Functional Assessment of Communication Skills (ASHA FACS)

"Rules of engagement" and client opportunities in our groups are based largely on FCT. Defined by Aten et al.

[2] as "any therapeutic endeavor that seeks to improve the patient's reception, processing, interacting socially, and expressing current physical and psychological needs," FCT uses any communication channel that provides an opportunity for the client to write or gesture to replace or augment language.

Scenarios of sessions are guided by Audrey Holland's functional end-points in aphasia treatment (Table 5-1) [3]. Given the present and future reality that few treatment sessions will be approved in a managed care climate, what skills should be addressed? The end-points are valuable everyday activities that can make the largest impact on safety and social well-being. Many of these end-points are based on functional behaviors listed in the ASHA FACS [4] and the Communicative Effectiveness Index [5].

The heart of the program described here, from assessment to treatment planning and program evaluation, is the ASHA FACS. It was designed to provide a "reliable, valid and practical tool for assessing functional communication" [6]. It was built on the framework of the World Health Organization's international classification as a functional measure to supplement tools that also define impairment and handicap [7]. Although the FACS did not become available until late 1995, I discovered it at the 1994 ASHA convention. The content appeared to fit our plan of care. The 43 behaviors, rated under four domains—social communication; communication of basic needs; daily planning; and reading, writing, and numbers—matched or approximated topics in our group and individual sessions. In fact, on viewing the list of FACS behaviors, staff found the areas relatively similar to functional short-term goals already in use with clients.

ENTRY CRITERIA

Referral mechanisms for speech-language pathology services vary from facility to facility and state to state. Ideally, the speech-language pathologist in an SNF screens all new admissions either by chart review or brief interview. This is not cost effective in a subacute setting, however, where the majority of admissions are for treatment of orthopedic or wound care.

The program described in this chapter came from an acute model in which we maintained the policy of screening by all disciplines for all new subacute admissions. Any clients with rehabilitative potential are immediately identified and considered for group treatment. Long-term care residents are also screened at admission. For long-standing residents, referral is made if the attending physician or nursing, or rehabilitation staff identifies a change in communication status or when notice is given that the individual has more potential than has been observed in daily living activities.

All clients with aphasia who demonstrated potential for restoration of communicative function are scheduled for the aphasia group. Exceptions are made only for those with severely decreased physical tolerance or cognitive deficits; however, these individuals are at times introduced for a short series of diagnostic sessions to assess further their potential to benefit from a group. Clients with chronic aphasia, referred for re-evaluation, might also be scheduled for a few sessions to assist in identifying strengths and approaches to maintaining skills in a long-term care setting (i.e., functional maintenance therapy).

ASSESSMENT

Subacute patients are first evaluated in a session lasting 45 minutes to 1 hour to determine:

- Communication diagnosis and prognosis
- Strengths and weaknesses
- Ability to use compensatory strategies
- Methods to teach staff and family effective communication strategies

The assessment process is also used to identify hidden capacities that can be used to maximize a client's successful participation in group and life situations. This is accomplished through both formal and informal test procedures.

Given the emphasis in the subacute setting on rapid identification of problems and approaches, two aphasia batteries have been found most beneficial: the Aphasia Diagnostic Profile (ADP) [8] and the Boston Assessment of Severe Aphasia (BASA) [9]. Both tests are helpful in defining impairments and identifying compensatory strategies that can be used to facilitate successful responses based on the principles of FCT. The BASA assists greatly with the severely affected client, especially when the task is to assess hidden strengths in severely impaired individuals with aphasia. Test items elicit responses to both linguistic and nonlinguistic information. Observations can be made of patient responses to contextual cues, vocal intonation, visual-spatial tasks, emotionally charged content, gestures, and melody. The test provides scaled scores and a quantification of verbal and gestural responses. The "singing" subtest also provides observation of the client's success in responding to melodic patterns or singing to optimize success in the aphasia group.

We administer the ADP to all other clients. During the test, nonlinguistic modes of communication are sought that may benefit group planning. Use of gestures is observed directly in the elicited gestures subtest and indirectly in the naming task because all pictured objects can be described through gestures. The ADP provides a profile of the patient's cognitive style, strategies, and compensatory behaviors.

For higher-level clients, we supplement the ADP with the 10-item functional reading subtest of the Reading Comprehension Battery of Aphasia [10]. This 10-item sample provides a good variety of brief, functional reading tasks and assists clinicians in judging competency for the evaluation report and the planning of the aphasia group. In the Communicative Abilities in Daily Living (CADL) [11], Holland provides a set of context-based interview questions and answers that taps a variety of strategies showing communicative competence.

In earlier days, I created a checklist from the first CADL [11] categories to use in groups. Staff members circle behaviors on a checklist as patients with aphasia respond to contextual cues. Group sessions are designed to promote strengths in role playing; social conventions; speech acts; divergencies; use of context; deixis; sequential relationships; nonverbal symbols; reading, writing, and calculations; and humor, metaphor, and absurdity. These CADL categories provide a way to assess strategy use. Strategies can be observed in a comprehensive, transdisciplinary setting, but in the "fast-forward" time frame of managed care, a more compact observation is needed. In addition, CADL-2 [12] has improved and streamlined the original format. Although the initial assessment addresses communicative modalities and some alternative methods, functional assessment is still needed. The ASHA FACS is rated after three contacts with the client. Sufficient observations for completing the ASHA FACS are obtained through aphasia group activities and in interviews with family and caregivers.

TREATMENT GOALS

We rarely find a reason to differentiate individual from group therapy goals. When I was first introduced to the ASHA FACS, I presented the FACS behaviors to my staff and requested that they begin using them as short-term goals as often as possible. Team members and case managers responded favorably to the department's move from focus on linguistic elements to more naturalistic events.

Initially, long-term goals were stated as a total FACS score indicating the level of communicative independence. For example, "(At discharge), the patient will achieve functional communicative independence with ___ (no/minimal/moderate/maximum) assistance, as measured by a total score of ___ on the ASHA FACS." Short-term goals were based on targeted behaviors in each domain. This worked well in that excellent functional objectives were written. However, when rehabilitation departments were asked to condense, streamline, and present 1-month goals for a care plan packet, we presented the following 1-month goals as progress toward independence in ASHA FACS domains:

- Communicate social needs with ___ assistance, as measured by a score of ___ on that domain of the ASHA FACS.
- Communicate basic needs with ___ assistance, as measured by a score of ___ on that domain of the ASHA FACS.
- Perform reading, writing, and number activities with ___ assistance, as measured by a score of ___ on that domain of the ASHA FACS.
- Perform activities of daily planning with ___ assistance, as measured by a score of ___ on that domain of the ASHA FACS.

Objectives to work toward these goals are selected from the list of behaviors under each FACS domain and expanded into specific settings by use of Leila Hartley's

TABLE 5-2.
Examples of Hartley Functional Communication Goals

Domain I: Home
    Personal health care and safety
    Family life and social interaction
    Use of memory aids and orientation
    Indoor leisure activities
    Housekeeping and maintenance
    Meal planning and preparation
    Use of telephone
    Spoken or written messages
    Correspondence
    Use of newspaper
    Child care
Domain II: Community
    Mobility
    Community safety
    Shopping
    Budgeting and banking
    Other community activities
    Medical care
    Making independent living arrangements
    Citizen advocate
Domain III: Work
    Job-seeking skills
    General job skills

Source: Adapted from LL Hartley. Cognitive-Communicative Abilities following Brain Injury: A Functional Approach. San Diego: Singular Publishing Group, 1995;266–271.

functional communication goals. Hartley [13] provides a six-page list of functional goals set in the domains of home, community, and work that fit well with the ASHA FACS behaviors (Table 5-2).

The majority of Hartley's functional communication goals can be easily merged with the ASHA FACS. Table 5-3 identifies 10 possible objectives, listed under family life and social interactions, leisure activities, and child care, which fit the FACS item "explaining how to do something."

DOCUMENTATION OF TREATMENT PROGRESS

The mechanism for tracking level of independence observed during group sessions is a simple grid (Figure 5-1) that lists the ASHA FACS behaviors by domain and allows space for scoring each group member. The grid is also used to collect data from individual sessions. When I complete a lesson plan for a group on the word processor, I insert a listing of the ASHA FACS behaviors and then select items that are observed in that lesson. For instance, 11 FACS behaviors are identified in the format planned for a lesson on calling 911 (Figure 5-2).

These lesson plans are printed out, distributed to staff and students as training materials, and kept in a department notebook for future use. Data are collected on the grid using any method that is comfortable for the observer: percentage, Porch Index of Communicative Abilities scoring, or a numbered (1–7) rating. The sheets are copied for the clinicians responsible for each patient and are incorporated into progress notes along with data

collected in individual sessions. We do not distinguish group from individual goals; however, when performance is particularly enhanced in one setting, scores may be reported separately and an interpretation offered. Progress notes are written weekly for subacute patients, as are measures of ASHA FACS behaviors targeted in the plan of care. The FACS domains selected as short-term goals are rated again at the time of the target date.

CLINICAL TECHNIQUES

Grouping aphasic clients by severity of impairment is optimal, but facility size and patient mix may limit the number of people with left hemisphere strokes and require grouping of severely affected and high-level clients together. Groups typically consist of two to six clients. A therapist-coach assists individuals in general, and severe patients in particular, during the first 2 weeks of treatment. If a well-established group consists of individuals at a similar level, new individuals with too mild or severe an impairment have group participation deferred until suitable cohorts are admitted. Groups meet 5 days a week for 45-minute sessions. Approximately 5–10 minutes of each session are spent in gathering the group and allowing spontaneous socialization before a topic is established. Five minutes are used at the end of the session to recap and bring closure to the activity.

The heart of the session is a well-planned, task-oriented activity that promotes a functional skill. To select the skill common to most of the group, we engage in a self-rating discussion based on the ASHA FACS. Each FACS behavior

TABLE 5-3.
Example of Merging ASHA FACS Behaviors and Hartley Functional Communication Goals

FACS domain: Social communication
FACS behavior: Explain how to do something
Hartley domain: Home
    Family life and social interactions:
    • Expresses unfamiliar task or chore to others
    • Gives directions to house or apartment to someone coming to visit
    Leisure activities—indoors:
    • Explains how to play a game or conduct activity to a family member or friend
    Child care:*
    • Teaches child how to handle emergencies
    • Explains desired behavior to a child
    • Explains new task or chore to child with supporting nonverbal communication
    • Gives directions for a game
    • Teaches child nutrition
    • Gives clear step-by-step directions
    • Explains to a child about safety

ASHA FACS = American Speech-Language-Hearing Association Functional Assessment of Communication Skills.
*These goals can be adapted to care of a spouse.
Source: Adapted from C Frattali, C Thompson, A Holland, et al. Functional Assessment of Communication Skills for Adults. Rockville, MD: American Speech-Language-Hearing Association, 1995; LL Hartley. Cognitive-Communicative Abilities following Brain Injury: A Functional Approach. San Diego: Singular Publishing Group, 1995;266–271.

Social Communication	Names/Scores					
Refers to familiar people by name						
Participates in group conversations						
Understands television and radio						
Expresses agreement and disagreement						
Explains how to do something						
Requests information						
Exchanges information on phone						
Answers yes-or-no questions						
Understands facial expression						
Understands tone of voice						
Follows simple verbal directions						
Understands intent						
Smiles or laughs at light-hearted . . .						
Understands nonliteral meaning						
Understands conversation in noisy . . .						
Initiates conversation with other people						
Adds new information on topic						
Changes topic in conversation						
Adjusts to change in topic						
Recognizes own communication errors						
Corrects own communication errors						

FIGURE 5-1.   **Example of score sheet to track ASHA FACS behaviors for the social communication domain. (ASHA FACS = American Speech-Language-Hearing Association Functional Assessment of Hearing Skills.)**

is stated in the first person (e.g., "I can explain how to do something"). Given the possibility of members' serious limitations in working memory, we reduce the self-rating to three choices: always, partly, and never. Three to five sessions are used to answer these questions one at a time and to discuss daily experiences, gripes, and triumphs in each area. We find that group veterans do not mind reassessment; they often give information about their advancement in quality of life. Although it is not easily quantified, a difference in tone of voice and facial expression is detectable when an individual has moved from despair and failure to increased self-confidence in the group.

Self-rating helps families to define losses objectively and to participate in setting priorities. Using such practical examples of family and rehabilitative life encourages reality checks and client and family control of their own program. Treatment tasks are selected from needs identified in the initial ASHA FACS rating. When first blending the ASHA FACS into the group format, I discovered that my notebook of group lesson plans fit quite well. Holland's end-points also were a good organizational framework for my files.

Another category that influences the choice of topics in aphasia group is survival skills. Communicating symptoms to medical, nursing, or therapy staff and reinforcing other disciplines' goals contribute to the health and safety of the patient (Table 5-4).

Targeting survival skills also identifies the speech-language pathologist as a team player and demonstrates a clear need for our in-patient services. Such skills overlap with the end-points. Clinicians need to target these survival skills for individuals returning to a lower level of care, particularly in an acute or subacute setting. Table 5-5 shows an example of a session using survival skills, and Figure 5-2 provides a score sheet for the session.

Well-planned sessions are a key factor in producing successful communicative exchanges during group. Two staff members are assigned to each group. All department staff rotate through a group assignment to become familiar with the format. In addition, all graduate students are assigned to groups. The second staff person is released to other responsibilities when a student is present on a rotation. Staff meet weekly to plan each week's group and to

ASHA FACS Behaviors	Names/Scores					
Social communication						
Participates in group conversations						
Exchanges information on phone						
Answers yes-or-no questions						
Follows simple verbal directions						
Adds new information on topic						
Communication of basic needs						
Requests help						
Makes needs and wants known						
Responds in an emergency						
Dials telephone numbers						
Reading, writing, and number concepts						
Understands environmental signs						
Understands printed material						

FIGURE 5-2. **Sample score sheet for 911 lesson plan. (ASHA FACS = American Speech-Language-Hearing Association Functional Assessment of Hearing Skills.)**

discuss any problems a patient may have exhibited during the previous week's group meeting.

Students from other disciplines and family members are assigned coaching or interactive roles in the group whenever possible. We also encourage staff from other departments to participate in the group. Although attendance by professional staff may be unrealistic, nursing, physical therapy (PT), and occupational therapy (OT) departments send students to observe the groups regularly. These visitors are invited to lend their expertise to the topic at hand. They often return to their departments raving about the aphasics' communication abilities and the relevance of the aphasia group, begging their supervisors to allow further participation. They also recognize the support we give to their disciplines by providing quality care through better communication. Observation of group sessions often results in a more transdisciplinary approach to functional communication than that used previously by speech-language pathologists and other therapists. The integration of clients' physical therapy goals is a high priority in group sessions. This is done in several ways:

- PT staff members are asked to define clients' safety "rules of the road." These definitions are repeated in every session.

- We assist PT staff in simplifying their language to improve client comprehension and compliance.
- PT and OT sessions are videotaped (with client permission) and viewed during the group meeting.

Survival skills are interspersed into other group meetings for sheer pleasure. I have collected a large number of videotapes with simplified story grammar, plausible information, humor and absurdity, and visual-spatial content to provide an esthetic, affectionate, or interesting experience worth sharing with a loved one or cohort (see Appendix 5-1). Videotapes with no or limited speech (e.g., silent movies) assist the client in encoding information without being penalized by linguistic limitations. In groups, I use 5- to 10-minute videotape segments with a preview-view-discuss format. Because the tapes illustrate many ways of communicating, nonverbal means of communicating content become more accessible. To accommodate high- and low-level clients in the same group, the videotaped segments are analyzed in the following manner:

- The story is broken into events or episodes with a limited number of information units (5–10 minutes).
- Story grammar is analyzed to identify setting, protagonists, events, and so on to prime group members with key vocabulary, gestures, or drawings.

TABLE 5-4.
Safety and Health Survival Skills

These suggested topics for group lesson plans involving safety and health address the following functional end-points:
- Signal and get help in an emergency
- Demonstrate retained competencies that are masked by aphasia
- Assert autonomy and independence, if not of action, at least of thought and opinion
- Follow simple instructions

Take Your Medicine: demonstrate competence to self-medicate: use medicine cups and pills to demonstrate ability to follow dosage; read prescriptions; discuss reasons for medications; assert self in discussion with doctor or nurse regarding continued needs

High Blood Pressure: understand foods and lifestyles; visit from nursing students to take blood pressure; discuss results

Talking to Your Doctor and Nurse: give symptoms verbally or non-verbally; indicate location and degree of pain; match symptoms to diseases

Visiting the Dentist: give symptoms; ask questions; anticipate events; rehearse visit

Visiting the Eye Doctor: practice variety of vision tests; process language style of examination directions and questions

You and Your Physical Therapist: take questionnaire to promote discussion; review language of physical therapy session; view and discuss videotaped physical therapy session of one group member; have physical therapy students observe for problem solving; have those with aphasia give adequate directions to speech-language pathologist on how to transfer them per plan of care

Emergency: discuss safety in the home; call 911; explain emergency event; sequence events when paramedic arrives; give reasons and steps if cardiopulmonary resuscitation is needed; understand "do not resuscitate" orders

Nurse!: discuss and practice when and how to gain attention of nurses and certified nursing assistants

---

- The tapes are shown once to the group without interruption or interpretation to allow events to be discussed in context and enjoyed.
- We review the tapes with a game or question-and-answer format to consolidate facts.

DISCHARGE CRITERIA

Patients remain in group therapy as long as they are rehabilitation candidates and want to participate. Discharge from group normally occurs when the patient is returning home or transferring to another facility. Patients who move to long-term care beds continue in group and individual treatment as long as they are making gains in communication. Group members are also discharged if they refuse or resist attending group. Such individuals are rare. Some may never have felt comfortable in groups. Others have comorbid factors, such as psychiatric problems, or are overwhelmed by their disability despite one-to-one coaching. Because these clients are often poor candidates for individual treatment, they are encouraged to attempt group therapy so that their strengths can be assessed in a more cost-effective manner when designing a maintenance program.

REIMBURSEMENT ISSUES

Fee structure for groups in the subacute setting is not directly considered; patients receive services based on their assessed needs. They are admitted under Medicare Part A or commercial insurance with an all-inclusive rate. Focus is placed on each client's clinical needs and the communicative modalities needed to achieve functional outcomes. Administration uses the statistics of group attendance in the annual cost report to Medicare, which contributes indirectly to determining rates. When clients make the transition to long-term care, billing is done via Medicare Part B, commercial insurance, or private pay, depending on the admission agreement.

Medicare intermediaries are highly inconsistent on reimbursement for group therapy. The fiscal intermediary for Medicare Part A in Syracuse, New York, provided the following guidelines (correspondence from Professional Relations Specialist, Medicare Part A, Syracuse, NY, to speech-language pathologist, Long Beach Memorial Hospital, Long Beach, NY, 1995):

- A speech-language pathologist must be present in each group session.
- Groups should be small (three to four members, or up to six members, is considered reasonable).
- Clear goals, objectives, and treatments for a specific patient must be in the medical record.
- The patient must have an individualized care plan.
- Progress notes must show a specific patient's participation and progress.

The group structure described in this chapter clearly falls within these guidelines. Admission and discharge criteria are based on rehabilitation potential and resulting outcomes.

TABLE 5-5.
Sample Lesson Plan: Calling 911 for Help

Objectives: Client will dial 911 and state name, location, agency needed, and problem.
1. Establish topic: group discussion of past experiences, availability of 911 in their counties, alternative numbers.
2. Collect list of various emergencies that could be reported to police, fire department, or ambulance (write on board) under each category.
3. Define the communication skills necessary to complete a call successfully.
4. Practice components: dialing 911; stating name, location, agency needed, and problem.
5. Have each patient practice a complete call.
6. Evaluate strengths and weaknesses; coach in the use of strategies that would increase effectiveness of the call.
7. Repeat the call with use of strategies.
Adaptation for low-level clients:
1. Have their turn last, after observing several models.
2. Narrow objective to dialing 911 or "O" and shouting "Help."
3. Have them select the symbol of the agency they would like to practice calling.
4. Have them select an emergency from a printed list (field narrowed to their level) or pick "out of a hat."
5. If group is well established, have them hand the phone to a high-level patient to complete call.
Materials needed: Telephone; symbols for fire, police, and ambulance; list of emergencies to add to choices if few are given

CONCLUSION

As a profession, we have been slow to translate what we know about communication into clear examples of how our clients' lives change. As a supervisor, I found novice clinicians challenged and willing to adopt a functional or pragmatic approach to aphasia therapy, but they often asked, "Does it ever get easier?" As a team, we learned to adopt the ASHA FACS domains and behaviors as our conceptual framework. After a relatively short period, we are able to answer that therapy does get easier with the ASHA FACS, and these guidelines make sense to all involved in the recovery of the individual with aphasia.

The ASHA FACS method is a coherent and productive guide in planning functional recovery from aphasia for both the clinician and consumer because it accomplishes the following:

- Identifies functional behaviors required to obtain communicative independence
- Provides a menu for establishing functional short-term and long-term goals
- Serves as a prompt in designing aphasia group activities
- Translates easily into a tracking mechanism of individual performance in the group
- Provides a sensitive, reliable measure of progress
- Communicates client's progress to fellow workers, administrators, and third-party payers in tangible terms
- Satisfies clients, families, and clinicians that group activities are both goal-driven and based on daily needs

REFERENCES

1. Groark CM. The Subacute Transition. Continuing Care Connection (Albany, NY: Healthcare Association of New York) Mar 1993, no. 15.
2. Aten J. Functional Communication Treatment. In R Chapey (ed), Language Intervention Strategies in Adult Aphasia. Baltimore: Williams & Wilkins, 1986;266–276.
3. Holland A. Functional end points. Presented at the Conference on Aphasia Treatment: Clinical Effectiveness in the New Health Care Environment, Cortland, NY, 1996.
4. Frattali C, Thompson C, Holland A, et al. Functional Assessment of Communication Skills for Adults. Rockville, MD: American Speech-Language-Hearing Association, 1995.
5. Lomas J, Pickard L, Bester S, et al. The communicative effectiveness index: development and psychometric evaluation of a functional communication measure for adult aphasia. J Speech Hear Disord 1989;54:113–124.
6. Frattali C, et al. American Speech-Language-Hearing Association Functional Assessment of Communication Skills—A Functional Outcome Measure for Adults. Rockville, MD: ASHA, 1995;41–46.
7. World Health Organization. International Classification of Impairments, Disabilities, and Handicaps. Geneva, Switzerland: WHO, 1980.
8. Helm-Estabrooks N. Aphasia Diagnostic Profiles Manual. Chicago: Riverside, 1992;11.
9. Helm-Estabrooks N, et al. Boston Assessment of Severe Aphasia Manual. Chicago: Riverside, 1989.
10. LaPointe L, Horner J. Reading Comprehension Battery for Aphasia. Tigard, OR: CC Publications, 1979.
11. Holland A. The Communicative Abilities in Daily Living: A Test of Functional Communication for Aphasic Adults. Austin, TX: Pro-Ed, 1980.
12. Holland A, Frattali C, Fromm D. The Communicative Abilities in Daily Living (revised). Austin, TX: Pro-Ed. (In press.)
13. Hartley LL. Cognitive-Communicative Abilities following Brain Injury: A Functional Approach. San Diego: Singular Publishing Group, 1995;266–271.

Appendix 5-1

MOVIE AND TELEVISION PROGRAM VIDEOS

These television programs and videotapes were selected for their high reliance on nonverbal information.

COMMERCIAL VIDEOTAPES

Adventures of Milo and Otis (Columbia Tristar Home Video; 76 minutes). Narrated adventures of a kitten and pug puppy, with multiple episodes that can be viewed in small segments.

Silent Movie, with Mel Brooks (Fox Video; 88 minutes). Slapstick with repetitive theme, absurdities, physical comedy, gestural communication, facial expressions.

Snowman, with Raymond Briggs (Columbia Tristar Home Video; 29 minutes). Animated fantasy with lovely music and no speech.

TELEVISION PROGRAMS

Jack Hanna's Animal Adventures (Web site: http://www.jackhanna.com; tel. 1-800-869-6789). Full of humor and great variety, these programs provide a wealth of material. There is an outstanding range of appeal for animal lovers, adventurers, travelers, and human interest.

Martha Stewart's Living (http://www.marthastewart.com). Excellent for procedural discourse; slow, relaxed pace; familiar procedures with her special twist; great material for describing similarities and differences; gardening segments appeal to both men and women.

Best of Saturday Night Live (Starmaker NBC Video, distributed by Anchor Bay Entertainment, 500 Kirsz Blvd, Troy, MI, 48084). Best appreciated by younger audiences. The opening skit is usually timely.

Your New House (Web site: http://www.yournewhouse.com; tel. 1-800-TOBUILD). Short and long how-to improvements or repairs on new and old homes are illustrated weekly. Printed transcripts are available via the Internet.

"Father Goose," *20/20* segment (Resolution, ABC News, P.O. Box 2284, S. Burlington, VT, 05407;1-800-913-3434). A superb, simple narrative that blends music, emotion, and visual imagery in a true story that was the basis of the movie *Fly Away Home*.

CHAPTER SIX

Aphasia Group Communication Treatment: The Aphasia Center of California Approach

Ellen Bernstein-Ellis and
Roberta J. Elman

PHILOSOPHY OF PROGRAM

The Aphasia Center of California (ACC) opened its doors as a nonprofit organization in September 1996. Founded by Roberta J. Elman, we were the first independent 501(c)(3) organization dedicated to providing direct services to individuals with aphasia. Our aphasia groups began in 1994, when the National Easter Seal Research Program funded our study to investigate the efficacy of group communication treatment for aphasia. The results of the study were positive [1]. Both statistical and anecdotal data told us that the establishment of the ACC would allow us to offer a greatly needed service to adults with aphasia and their caregivers. Guided by our mission statement—to encourage and expand communication skills and maximize psychosocial well-being for those with aphasia—we launched the ACC with an all-volunteer staff of certified speech-language pathologists. Housed in a senior center in Oakland, California, we currently offer six ongoing conversation groups, a caregiver's support group, several reading and writing groups, and an art class co-facilitated by the Adult Education Department of the local school district. We are committed to providing the treatment array that our members feel best serves their interests and needs [2]. In response to participant requests, we plan to offer a computer skills class and to support other recreational activities.

Several factors converged to forge the philosophic foundation of the ACC. First, we felt the urgent need to develop a viable, effective model for providing aphasia treatment under the changes in health care provision and reimbursement. Due to the emergence of managed care, our treatment environment dramatically changed. The number of visits authorized by insurance carriers shrank. The nature of aphasia was not changing, but the time available to treat communication deficits was, and this reduction had serious implications. It was becoming the norm for a patient who would have received a 3- to 6-month treatment authorization to have only six to 10 authorized visits [3]. This forced a significant restructuring of our treatment goals and priorities [4].

We struggled with many questions about the impact of managed care on our clinical approach. What type of communication goals could be met in the course of 10 sessions? Which goals would have the greatest impact on a patient's quality of life at the end of this brief clinical contact [4]? What treatment techniques and approaches, many of which developed based on lengthy treatment trials, would be effective in a much-abbreviated clinical trial? Patients who recognized that they would benefit from additional treatment often did not have the financial resources to pursue private-pay options. Although we still valued individual treatment for aphasia, we decided to consider lower-cost but efficacious options for meeting the needs of our clients.

Another primary factor in the formation of the ACC was our conscious decision to consider aphasia a chronic disorder [2]. Regardless of whether stroke survivors with aphasia had 10 therapy sessions or 50, many were left with significant and lasting residual deficits [5–8]. Even clients with mild aphasia told us that the onset of aphasia imposed lifelong changes in their communicative abilities [3]. We considered aphasia to be like any other chronic medical condition in which full recovery to premorbid status was unlikely [2]. For instance, with the onset of diabetes, ongoing insulin treatment may be needed to manage the condition. It would not be ethical to withdraw insulin after an arbitrary period without substituting another treatment. Is it surprising that some stroke survivors become isolated and depressed after discharge from speech-language therapy? What should we do to replace the support and value that the therapeutic environment once provided? Diabetic patients are not "discharged" from the treatment designed to manage their chronic disorder. We concluded that patients with chronic aphasia deserved the same conceptual approach of ongoing management to support their communication impairment.

Health club membership may be a useful analogy for the sustained management of aphasia. People have many reasons for joining a health club, such as improving their level of fitness or attempting weight reduction. When the goal is achieved, the patron is not asked to leave the club. Rather, they are encouraged to continue their participation to sustain their accomplishment. The benefit of the exercise does not diminish once the goal is met. Some people continue to make improvements in their fitness level and actually exceed their original goal. Continued health club membership may enhance the chances that a person will maintain the gains that he or she made.

Like health club members, each member of an aphasia treatment group has a persisting condition. Management of the condition may be enhanced by group treatment sessions that facilitate the use of strategies to optimize communication. Participating in weekly or biweekly "workouts" that promote successful communicative interactions may help sustain gains made in individual therapy. Some members make new gains over time due to the exposure to new strategies via peer modeling, the opportunity for practice and feedback, and the psychosocial support offered by the group environment. Thus, membership in an aphasia center can have ongoing benefits.

This sustained management approach is consistent with the model provided by the World Health Organization (WHO) in the *International Classification of Impairments, Disabilities, and Handicaps* (ICIDH) [9]. Such a model demonstrates that we should address not only the linguistic deficits of aphasia but also the resulting disabilities and handicaps. The proposed WHO revisions (ICIDH-2) update this triad to impairment, activity, and participation, which appear even more closely aligned with the ACC's sustained management approach to the treatment of aphasia. The ICIDH-2 "attempts to provide a synthesis that offers a coherent view of different dimensions of health at both biological and social levels" [10]. The new proposed model is seen as both interactional and dynamic; it recognizes the complex relationships between the health condition and environmental and personal factors. If the proposed changes are adopted, the revised WHO model will likely have a significant impact on the treatment of many health conditions, including those affecting speech and language.

We have learned that some very valuable treatment goals may take much longer to achieve than our training taught us to expect. We also have learned that our members with aphasia make gains after the standard recovery periods [1,11]. In forming the ACC, we wanted to provide an environment that would support the ongoing improvement that many individuals with aphasia are capable of making over time. Our members and their families have told us about personal successes that significantly affect quality of life that they attribute, at least in part, to participation in our groups. Through their stories, we have learned that our members make changes and achieve goals that are not always captured by performance on standardized speech and language assessment tools but are nonetheless a vital contribution to their adjustment to living with aphasia.

A final factor was strongly responsible for the creation of the ACC. A 1989 visit to the Aphasia Centre–North York in Toronto, Canada, greatly influenced our perspective of aphasia groups. The treatment model we saw was a source of clinical motivation and inspiration [12–14]. Its impact has also been cited by other clinical visitors [15–17].

ENTRY CRITERIA

After completing our study on the efficacy of group therapy for aphasia [1], we opened our program to the community at large. Currently, the ACC allows any adult with aphasia to attend. People travel to our groups from six counties in the San Francisco–Oakland Bay Area, and some come from more than 60 miles away. The primary etiology of our group members is either thromboembolic or hemorrhagic stroke. Some members have had only a single documented cerebrovascular incident. Others have a history of multiple strokes. We accept all levels of aphasia severity. Some members have less common etiologies, such as primary progressive aphasia, brain abscess, chemotherapy-induced aphasia, and unknown etiologies. As long as the behavioral characteristics are "aphasia-like" and other behaviors do not detract from participation, an individual is welcome to join. Although we do not accept someone with a primary diagnosis of dementia, some of our members are coping with varying degrees of cognitive decline.

There is no entry criterion for time post-onset. Our members range from 1 month post-stroke to more than 20 years post-stroke. The majority of our members are from 3 months to 10 years post-onset. We have a variety of referral sources. Some members locate us through the local newspaper, either from a feature story about the ACC or from a community bulletin board listing. Other members come via referral from local speech-language pathologists at hospitals, outpatient therapy clinics, or from private practices. Others hear about the ACC through their personal grapevine of information, including friends, the National Aphasia Association, our Web site, or our community outreach projects.

ASSESSMENT

During the research phase of our groups, we completed a standard battery of quantitative and qualitative measures of speech-language performance and psychosocial status on every member. Once we became an independent nonprofit organization, we did not have the resources to complete these assessments as standard practice. We now gather relevant information through several sources. Usually, we interview either the potential member or her caregiver by telephone. Frequently, we are able to talk directly with the previous speech-language therapist. These contacts allow us to obtain medical background, personal and social information, and treatment history and to glean a sense of communicative functioning across the modalities. Sometimes we can obtain records with relevant assessment information. When we have the services of a student intern, we try to arrange for a supervised assessment session. We select members for whom we feel that the information from a standard aphasia battery would help us to better understand their communication profiles.

Once an individual is interested in attending our program, we choose a group for that potential member to observe, based on which of our groups have an opening and the person's schedule. In addition, we consider how a person's functioning and personality might interact with the current composition of the group. Sometimes, due to logistical constraints, there is simply no choice of group, but the groups are remarkably able to adapt to the diversity of their membership. The first observation session in the group allows us to assess informally the prospective participant's communicative and social style. Each member completes an emergency information form that provides personal contacts, pertinent medical history, and current medications. Group composition is addressed further under Clinical Techniques.

TREATMENT GOALS

As we began to formulate the types of groups to promote, our experience in Canada helped guide our treatment model. Our primary treatment goals are to enhance communication skills and maximize psychosocial well-being of individuals with aphasia. These primary goals are achieved by focusing on the following:

- *Member and family education.* We believe that people with aphasia and those who care about them benefit from understanding the nature of the communication disorder. Most of our stroke survivors and their families tell us that they had never heard the word *aphasia* until after their stroke. Very little or no patient education has been offered to most of our members before they come to the ACC. Many of our members have never met anyone else living with aphasia until they attend our groups, and they are grateful for the connection they feel.

- *Personal goals.* We try to promote an increased awareness of each member's personal goals and progress made toward those goals. We support attempts at communicative situations personally relevant to each member. We have found that many members find it difficult to acknowledge their gains and therefore benefit greatly from the recognition the group gives to them.

- *Conversational practice.* We firmly believe that the benefits of conversational practice cross all severity levels and types of aphasia. Experience has taught us that it typically takes more effort to promote cross-talk and member-led discussions in groups composed of members with moderate-to-severe aphasia, but there remains a natural motivation to share topics of mutual interest, regardless of severity level. Capobianco and Mahli [18] recognize the value of the group setting in that "patients congratulate each other, advise each other, and argue with each other—all of which are normal communication activities." When a group expresses an interest in any topic or theme, there is a communicative spark, which can then be fanned by choosing clinical techniques that promote interaction and information exchange. We view the topic or task as the springboard, rather than the vehicle, for sparking communicative intent. More often than not, an introduced topic has been cast aside to follow whatever unpredictable conversational path the group finds more interesting and thus more conversationally productive.

- *Communicative strategies.* We focus on improving the ability to convey a message using whatever strategy is most useful for that individual. Typically, our focus is on content exchange instead of linguistic accuracy. The clinician and group members model a variety of strategies to facilitate the successful exchange of information, including the use of communicative drawing, graphic supplementation, natural gestures, and environmental resources, such as maps, visual scales, calendars, photographs, and newspapers.

- *Conversational initiation.* We focus on increasing initiation in conversational exchanges. Davis and Wilcox [19,20] emphasize the importance of sharing the communicative burden in a conversation. Our clinical experience revealed that the aphasic partner typically assumes a more passive, responder role, whereas the nonaphasic partner becomes the initiator. This was particularly true of our clients with moderate-to-severe aphasia. Our groups focus on both the initiator and responder roles of the turn-taking process. We believe it is essential for the therapist to maximize the members' opportunity to direct the discussion. This is different from traditional didactic treatment models, which often place the primary responsibility for leading the group on the therapist.

- *Conversational cross-talk.* We promote *cross-talk*, or exchanges among group members. It is easy to fall into a tea-party or talk-show host pattern, where the exchanges bounce from the clinician to a member and then back to the clinician, who again initiates an exchange with another member. The goal is to encourage members to follow up on group member questions and to offer comments to one another.

These treatment goals required that we embark into new clinical territory. The skills needed to facilitate participant-shared groups were markedly different from those used to direct individual therapy sessions. Even after observing a successful group model at the Toronto center, we found it much more difficult than anticipated to make changes in our clinical style. As one student intern said,

> It looks so easy when I observe the group, but when I try to do it, I'm surprised at how hard it is. It's like when you are skiing down a hill and you see a rock straight ahead. You know you should avoid it, but for some reason you run straight into it. I know I need to change course with the group, but somehow I still head straight for that rock.

The clinical techniques described later should help guide other clinicians around at least a few of the clinical obstacles that we faced while learning to facilitate groups.

DOCUMENTATION OF PROGRESS

The challenge of providing services as a nonprofit organization with limited resources has left us unable to invest large amounts of time in formal reassessments. We occasionally use the services of student interns to retest members who have not been assessed recently. Informal conversations with members and their families allow us to track reports of changes in their communicative or psychosocial status. At staff meetings, we discuss changes observed during group sessions. Informal logs are helpful in tracking anecdotal information. We also keep interesting samples of communicative drawings to allow for comparison over time. We hope that with additional financial support, we will be able to invest more time in documenting progress. Part of the challenge lies in our interest in tools that provide meaningful information, including quality of life changes. Few tools are available that are appropriate for use with the aphasic population [21–23].

The following brief case study illustrates the outcomes of a rather typical ACC participant. J.B., a 48-year-old woman, suffered a hemorrhagic stroke that left her with a moderately severe nonfluent aphasia and right-sided paralysis. Unable to live independently, she lived with her parents. She started in our group approximately 6 months post-onset, after discharge from individual speech-language therapy. At entry into the program, J.B.'s interactions during group were slow and laborious. She needed constant coaching to use communicative strategies. Most notable was her poor eye contact. She spent most of the session looking down at the table. Initiation of communicative interactions was markedly impaired. She expressed frustration and depression over the loss of her job as a school bus driver, her loss of independence, and her loss of an active social schedule.

J.B. attended group once weekly. The group encouraged her to use graphic attempts and communicative drawing as strategies to help convey content. The clinician asked the group members to cue J.B. about her eye contact. Discussions often addressed the psychosocial issues with which she was struggling, and group members offered support, perspective, and experience. She began to implement some of the group's suggestions, starting with buying a wristwatch with large clear numbers and using a small notebook to track basic biographic and personal information. Over a 2-year period, her successful communicative attempts increased in phrase length and content. There was a noticeable improvement in her eye contact and social skills. She moved back into her own home and began living independently. J.B. learned how to take public transportation, which included giving instructions to the receptionist about her pickup schedule. She started an exercise class at a local YMCA. She also participated in a reading and writing class and an art class at the ACC.

It has been remarkable to watch J.B. emerge as a mentor to other aphasic participants in these classes. She began to take people under her wing and successfully introduced several new members to the public transportation system for disabled citizens. She became pivotal in group discussions for initiating cross-talk. She introduced new topics and would ask follow-up questions without prompting, and her eye contact was almost always appropriate.

J.B.'s rather remarkable improvement demonstrates what we have seen to varying degrees with many of our members. These observations have convinced us that "an individual with aphasia should not be expected to discontinue activities or groups that enhance socialization, conversation, and/or reintegration back into community activities through the reduction of communicative barriers" [2].

CLINICAL TECHNIQUES

Group Structure

Our groups are 90 minutes long. Typically, this includes a 15-minute overlap time between groups, during which members are encouraged to mix and converse. Most groups range in size from five to 10 members, with six to eight members preferred. Our experience has shown that it is difficult to keep the conversational ball rolling in groups of less than four members. With groups larger than 10 members, it may be difficult to give everyone ample time to participate. We have learned that there are no hard and fast rules about group composition. Rather, the clinician's personal preference should be the primary guide. Two of us prefer to form groups using severity as the lead attribute for placement. We put people with mild-to-moderate aphasia in one group and people with moderate-to-severe aphasia in another. Those with moderate aphasia often work well in either group. Grouping by severity seems to accommodate discussions about adjustment issues associated with the

severity of the communication disorder. Our groups with milder aphasia seem to appreciate the opportunity to have quicker-paced, philosophic discussions that members with a greater degree of aphasia may have trouble following. Another clinician at the ACC prefers to mix aphasia severity in her groups. She feels that this promotes modeling and coaching opportunities while enriching the variety of interactions within the group. We are convinced that either approach to forming groups works exceedingly well.

We have been asked if an individual with Wernicke's aphasia can benefit from a group setting. We indeed advocate integrating people with poor auditory comprehension into our groups. These people need to develop functional social conversation skills just as much as those with nonfluent aphasia. People with Wernicke's aphasia have different goals and benefit from different strategies, but they are excellent candidates for group membership. The group environment provides ample opportunity for practicing important skills, such as clarifying conversational input and learning to ask for multiple sources of input.

As group members enter the ACC's primary therapy room, the first order of business is to locate their name tags from the wall hanger, which boasts more than 70 names. Members wear name tags at every session to promote the use of names during conversational exchanges. Our groups provide a warm welcome to participants. There is a deliberate effort to greet everyone who comes in the door. Coffee and other beverages are distributed, usually by a group member who is willing to help with hospitality tasks. Family members are often busy greeting one another and talking with the clinician about relevant points of information. Once everyone is settled around the table, any guest for the day is introduced and handed a temporary name tag. We request that family members periodically observe, and we get a variety of other observers, including potential members and their families, graduate students, and other professionals. Our only rule regarding visitors is firm: They must join us around the table and participate as a group member. No one is allowed to sit back in the corner and watch us interact. This rule promotes a more natural conversational environment and provides novelty and variety in conversational partners. Group members are responsible for introductions and for getting to know the guests.

When the group is ready to start, we try to follow up on a conversational element from the previous week or get a sense of a topic that the group is interested in discussing. Our groups have evolved from having preplanned "themes" to having topical discussions, including whatever is most relevant to their interests that day. Looking back at our early philosophic discussions, we realized that relying on themes was our safety net. In the beginning, it felt too overwhelming to go into a group without some sort of structured clinical plan. Our best interactive, participatory discussions typically strayed far from the preplanned theme, so we learned that success did not rely on having a specific set of tasks or topics. Now, we rotate tasks or topics depending on day-to-day context. Some discussions are more structured than others, such as those addressing stroke education, role-playing communicative situations, interviewing guests, or sharing keepsakes or photos. Other discussions are less structured, such as those involving current events, personal activities, vacation or holiday plans, post-stroke adjustment discussions, and personal interests and hobbies. Our focus now is on the techniques needed to promote conversational initiation and facilitate the exchange of information regardless of the task or topic that emerges from the conversational menu.

Increasing Conversational Initiation

Increasing the conversational control and initiation of our members with aphasia is a primary goal of our groups. We have found various techniques useful for addressing this goal:

1. *Directing the facilitator's role to a specific group member, or "you're it."* This technique consists of asking a group member to lead the discussion about a specific topic. A peer facilitator can gather opinions about an upcoming election, survey each person's favorite type of pie, or inquire about everyone's weekend. This technique can be adapted across severity levels. Some members may need only a key word to help formulate a query, whereas others may benefit from a written script to prompt the question. Scripting refers to writing out anywhere from a few words to a full sentence and handing it to the member, who either reads it directly or uses it as a springboard [16]. Allowing the member to facilitate the discussion becomes particularly dynamic when the member in charge takes on an active role and goes beyond the question at hand. The group is at its best when the follow-up questions and feedback come from their peer facilitator rather than the clinician.

2. *Passing the question, or "passing the ball."* With this technique, the facilitator's role is shared around the table. The group discusses a certain topic and, as each person concludes a turn, he or she restates the question or topic for the next person. This method ensures that each member gets a turn to initiate and to respond. It helps to put the focus on the members instead of allowing a clinical "tea-party" pattern to develop between the clinician and the group members. This technique also lends itself to adaptation across severity levels. Mildly aphasic members may elaborate on the original question or theme as they "pass the ball," whereas nonverbal members may establish a communicative gesture to indicate that it is the next group member's turn.

3. *Address a member's participation level.* We ask, "Who hasn't had a turn yet?" or "Who's been too quiet?" This tactic works best when group members begin to monitor each other's participation level and try to ensure that everyone takes a turn.

4. *Request that members generate a topic.* We ask members to bring in news articles, personal items, photos, or anything of interest. We ask the group, "What do you want to talk about?" This promotes novelty and humor, both essential elements for successful groups. Our best groups are ones that share laughter. Frequently, it is a group member who first recognizes the humor in a situation or initiates a joke. The laughter they share crosses aphasia types and severity.

5. *Peer "scaffolding" or cueing.* The term *scaffolding* refers to the opportunity for one or more group members to help another group member around some sort of communicative block. Instead of the clinician providing a cue, the clinician asks, "Who can help Mrs. X get her message across?" This technique works well when several members offer help. By building on each other's attempts, members are able to clarify the message. The group recognizes that the message has been directed by the group and not the clinician.

6. *Encouraging peer feedback.* Frequently, group members do not allow someone to "bail out" when faced with a communicative block. Instead, group members display support by passing a pad of paper to encourage a drawing or writing attempt, or they hand another member their communication book, or request that the member slow down or speak louder. Members tell one another, "Yes, you can!" or "Try to do it," and these exchanges seem to have more impact coming from a peer than from the clinician.

7. *Peer volunteers.* We have asked mildly aphasic members to volunteer in our mild-to-moderate aphasia groups, and we have asked both mildly and severely aphasic members to volunteer in our moderate-to-severe aphasia groups. Volunteers are selected for their ability to model good communicative strategies or interactions. One of our most outstanding volunteers, L.I., has severely impaired auditory comprehension and verbal output limited to "Hey, mom!" However, he gleans contextual information and uses environmental resources very effectively. L.I. can link a long string of functional gestures or combine several communicative elements in a drawing to convey complex information. He frequently initiates conversational topics using these strategies. The group as a whole benefits from his modeling of gestures and drawings.

8. *Personalizing the discussion.* It is important to move from the key topic at hand to people's personal experiences or opinions about that topic. For instance, if a member brings up a news item about France, there is opportunity for a series of related questions, such as "Who has been to France?" "Who likes French cuisine?" or even "Did anyone see the movie *Gigi*?" Although the key topic can often hold the group's interest, sometimes it is the related questions that spark the real conversation.

Increasing Exchange of Information

Another primary goal of our groups is to facilitate exchange of information. We use several techniques for that purpose:

1. *Support the flow of ideas with graphic attempts or communicative drawing.* We frequently encourage members to draw or write to enhance their message. Pads of paper and pens are standard items on our table and are distributed to everyone in every group, regardless of severity. The clinician also uses drawing and graphics as a standard way to emphasize content or to confirm information. We often prompt members, "Can you draw or write it?" or "How else can you show me what you mean?" Members often exchange different ways of approaching a drawing and are usually delighted to offer a better version than the clinician's. Some members seem to have a natural affinity for drawing and, with support and guidance, use it very effectively. Others need a higher level of support, training, and modeling. It is beyond the scope of this chapter to review the skills needed for communicative drawing. Please refer to the work of Lyon [24] for a detailed description of this useful technique.

2. *Graphic choices.* In this technique, the clinician presents several viable responses to a member so that he can indicate the preferred choice [25]. For example, if we're discussing favorite cuisine, we might write "Mexican, French, Indian, Italian" in a blank column on a pad of paper and present it to members who are primarily nonverbal or who have severely impaired auditory comprehension. Letting members select the item themselves lets them take the lead in responding.

3. *Natural gestures.* During a conversation, we often ask, "How can you show me that?" Sometimes brief, simple gestures are sufficient, and other times more elaborate gestures help to convey the message. Again, group members often can generate a better way to show something than the clinician's model.

4. *Communicative resources.* We make sure that maps, newspapers, number lines, personalized notebooks, visual scales, photos, an illustrated dictionary, and calendars are always available. When members cannot remember the name of the movie they just saw, the movie section of the newspaper is nearby. When members cannot recall the name of the place they plan to go on vacation, the appropriate map is within arm's reach. We have laminated maps of our local area, the United States, and the world. When trying to determine how much a nonverbal member likes something, we use a laminated number line. There is a sad face over the number 1 and a happy face over the number 10. Our members carefully select where their response falls along the continuum. We also encourage our members to take matchbooks or business cards when they go to a restaurant as a way to show the group the restaurant's name. Using these items allows the members, instead of the clinician, to take the lead in providing information.

5. *Weekly activity highlights form.* Families are coached to summarize highlights in a special form (Figure 6-1) in addition to providing information about routines. A trip to the grocery store, a new outfit, or a weekly hair appointment can provide a tremendous amount of potential conversational material. Some members attempt to complete the information form themselves each week. For some, the form acts like a script and allows them to take the lead in sharing information with the group. For a nonverbal member, the form gives the clinician specific, personally relevant information that can be used to involve that member in the discussion. These forms provide a gateway to participation for members who are less able to initiate content or for members with a moderate-to-severe fluent aphasia.

Table 6-1 summarizes some of our best ways to spark dynamic conversation in aphasia groups.

Management Issues

Along with these helpful techniques, we have also learned some important management issues inherent in the group setting. One issue involves handling one or two group members who become overly dominant or egocentric. These members may occupy more than their fair share of the group's conversational time. They may not monitor their own turn taking. One solution is to ask that member to be in charge of making sure that everyone participates. We ask him to "help us to include every member of the group." Sometimes we are more directive and state that we need time for each person to respond.

The clinician is also at high risk for dominating the group. It is often hard for the clinician not to dominate by virtue of expertise. Although there is a definite tendency to jump in immediately and provide needed cues, it is important to learn to involve the group members in overcoming any communicative obstacles. The clinician needs to ask, "What can Mary do to get her message across?" or "Could someone show another way to draw an airplane?" or "Who can show us a way to gesture driving?" These methods all support increasing the members' participation while reducing the clinician's dominance. Kagan [12] refers to the high level of skill needed to unmask an aphasic member's competency. Beeson and Holland [16] define a "communication broker" as one who interprets, facilitates, and guides communicative exchanges among group members. The challenge lies in balancing these roles. It is crucial for the clinician to learn the difference between being a "communication broker" and overfacilitating.

When a clinician gives up tight control of the discussion's content, awkward or uncomfortable issues may come up. Racial, religious, political, sexual, and gender-related topics frequently generate strong feelings. It is absolutely essential to establish ground rules for group standards of behavior. We have agreed that individuals who openly promote bigoted racial or religious attitudes are not welcome in our groups. That is not to say that our members must agree on heated topics. One of the special

Name: _____   **Date:** _____

Please bring us up to date on events since our last meeting. This information helps us to include more about each member in our group discussions. Both routine and special events are of interest to us.

Visitors

Name of visitor   Relationship to Aphasia Center member

_____   _____

_____   _____

_____   _____

_____   _____

Activities

_____

_____

_____

_____

Anything else you'd like to add (e.g., upcoming events, other information)?

_____

_____

_____

_____

FIGURE 6-1.   **Aphasia Center of California weekly activity highlights form.**

TABLE 6-1.
Best Bets for Sparking Conversation with Aphasia Groups

Capitalize on the group's lead
   Beware of preset agendas or themes
   Allow the group to inform you
   Follow the group's interests
   Encourage peer feedback
Increase member participation
   Allow group members to facilitate
   Novelty promotes interest
   Resources assist participation
   Humor enriches and motivates

attributes of the ACC is the wide diversity of our group members in cultural, economic, professional, and educational backgrounds. Part of the success of our groups comes from the common bond that forms from sharing life with aphasia. Our differences make the discussions more interesting and dynamic, and our members share a deep respect and appreciation for one another.

A clinician must learn how to balance the techniques he or she chooses with the severity and size of the group. Some techniques are more labor intensive than others and may take too long in larger groups, where it is important to mon-itor the amount of time each person has to participate. It typically takes longer to communicate and confirm information with an aphasic conversational partner, which can impair the conversational flow. This may result in side conversations that detract from the main conversational focus. We try to let the group know when a member needs extra time to convey a message. We encourage the group to have patience. The clinician needs to bring the group back to a unified focus.

Facilitating participant-led groups provides additional challenges for the clinician. The clinician must understand the unique "flavor" of each group. Some groups like to discuss current events; others prefer psychosocial issues or social topics. Groups seem to flourish when the clinician can adjust to the group's preferences. It is important for group members to understand that it takes time to form group bonds and cohesiveness. This facilitates the acclimation process and promotes realistic expectations for new group members.

Another challenge is being sensitive to the appropriate yardstick of change for group members. An ongoing group for adults with chronic aphasia needs to focus beyond linguistic changes to those that affect the members' quality of life. It is important to understand the issues of impairment, activity, and participation in relation to aphasia. As we broaden our perspective on the impact of aphasia on the lives of the individual, the caregivers,

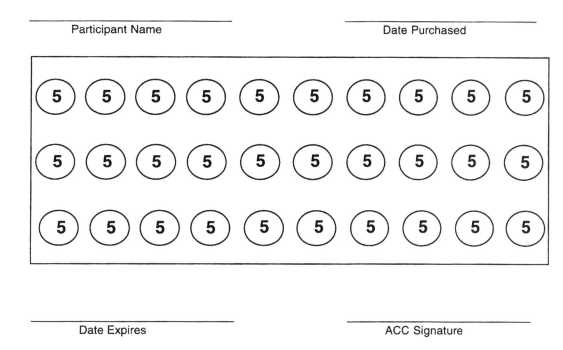

FIGURE 6-2.   **Aphasia Center of California session card.**

and the community, we need to find ways to acknowledge and track progress that represents meaningful change.

DISCHARGE CRITERIA

At the ACC, we do not believe in therapist-ordained discharge criteria. We consider aphasia a chronic disorder that deserves continued communication and psychosocial support for as long as desired. ACC participants self-determine the frequency and duration of their attendance. As Elman [2] has said, "rather than a therapist determining a discharge date, the individuals having aphasia determine whether they desire discharge from the program. And using a market-based system, they vote with their feet."

REIMBURSEMENT

We have chosen to seek the majority of reimbursement for our groups outside the traditional health care reimbursement system [2]. We depend primarily on private fees for our speech-language pathologist–facilitated groups. Participants who attend one group weekly pay $15 per session. Participants who elect to attend twice a week pay $10 for the second visit. People enroll in ACC groups by purchasing a $150 session card (Figure 6-2) that is kept at the center. They "spend down" this card as the therapist crosses off the cost at each session attended. The session card is composed of $5 circles, allowing the therapist to cross off $15 and $10 sessions on the same card. An additional advantage of this card system is that there is no need to schedule makeup sessions if participants are ill or have medical appointments. When all sessions on the card have been crossed off, participants

make a decision about re-enrollment. If they decide to continue in the groups, they purchase another $150 card. In addition to private payment directly from participants, several third-party payers are authorizing payment for our treatment groups.

Because the ACC is a charitable nonprofit organization, our board of directors and staff are committed to keeping program fees affordable. In addition, sliding fee reductions are available to those with low incomes, which permits everyone who can benefit to attend. Our recreational activities are co-facilitated by adult education instructors and are offered as a "value-added" service at no additional cost to current ACC participants.

CONCLUSION

The greatest rewards of the ACC come from the stories our group members and their families share with us about the impact the ACC has had on their adjustment to living with aphasia. These stories highlight new communicative successes and improvements in social adjustment. Most important, our members tell us that they feel connected to the ACC community and that this connection helps them to find greater meaning in their lives. As our group members help each other, they also help us to achieve a better understanding of what quality of life means, especially when living with aphasia.

REFERENCES

1. Elman RJ, Bernstein-Ellis EG. The efficacy of group communication treatment in adults with chronic aphasia. J Speech Lang Hear Res. (In press.)

2. Elman RJ. Memories of the "plateau": health care changes provide an opportunity to redefine aphasia treatment and discharge. Aphasiology 1998;12:227–231.

3. Elman RJ, Bernstein-Ellis EG. What is functional? Am J Speech Lang Pathol 1995;4:115–117.

4. Elman RJ. Aphasia treatment planning in an outpatient medical rehabilitation center: where do we go from here? Neurophysiology and Neurogenic Speech and Language Disorders Special Interest Division 2 Newsletter 1994;10:9–13.

5. Holland AJ. Some thoughts on future needs and directions for research and treatment of aphasia. NIDCD Monograph 1992;2:147–152.

6. Lyon JG. Communicative use and participation in life for aphasic adults in natural settings: the scope of the problem. Am J Speech Lang Pathol 1992;1:7–14.

7. Lyon JG. Coping with Aphasia. San Diego, CA: Singular Publishing Group, 1997.

8. Parr S, Byng S, Gilpin S, Ireland S. Talking about Aphasia: Living with Loss of Language after Stroke. Buckingham, UK: Open University Press, 1997.

9. World Health Organization. International Classification of Impairments, Disabilities, and Handicaps: A Manual for Classification Relating to the Consequences of Disease. Geneva, Switzerland: WHO, 1980.

10. World Health Organization. ICIDH-2 International Classification of Impairments, Activities, and Participation. [http://www.who.int/msa/mnh/ems/icidh/index.html]

11. Elman RJ, Bernstein-Ellis EG. Effectiveness of group communication treatment for individuals with chronic aphasia [abstract]. ASHA 1996;38:52.

12. Kagan A. Revealing the competence of aphasic adults through conversation: a challenge to health professionals. Top Stroke Rehabil 1995;2:15–28.

13. Kagan A, Gailey G. Functional Is Not Enough: Training Conversation Partners for Aphasic Adults. In AL Holland, MM Forbes (eds), Aphasia Treatment: World Perspectives. San Diego: Singular Publishing Group, 1993;199–225.

14. Kagan A, Winckel J, Shumway E. Pictographic Communication Resources. North York, Ontario: Aphasia Centre of North York, 1996.

15. Hersh D. Beyond the "plateau": discharge dilemmas in chronic aphasia. Aphasiology 1998;12:207–218.

16. Beeson PM, Holland AL. Aphasia Groups: An Approach to Long-Term Rehabilitation. Telerounds No. 19. Tucson, AZ: National Center for Neurogenic Communication Disorders, 1994.

17. Jordan L, Kaiser W. Aphasia: A Social Approach. London: Chapman & Hall, 1996.

18. Capobianco R, Mahli L. Senior Stroke Group: A Model for Educationally Based Group Treatment. Focus on Geriatric Care and Rehabilitation. Frederick, MD: Aspen Publishers, 1995;1–8.

19. Davis GA. Pragmatics and Treatment. In R Chapey (ed), Language Intervention Strategies in Adult Aphasia. Baltimore: Williams & Wilkins, 1986;251–265.

20. Davis GA, Wilcox MJ. Incorporating Parameters of Natural Conversation in Aphasia Treatment. In R Chapey (ed), Language Intervention Strategies in Adult Aphasia. Baltimore: Williams & Wilkins, 1981;169–193.

21. Frattali CM. Measuring disability. Neurophysiology and Neurogenic Speech and Language Disorders Special Interest Division 2 Newsletter 1996;12:7–10.

22. Frattali CM, Thompson CK, Holland AL, et al. American Speech-Language-Hearing Association Functional Assessment of Communication Skills for Adults. Rockville, MD: ASHA, 1995.

23. Simmons-Mackie N, Damico J. Accounting for handicaps in aphasia: communicative assessment from an authentic social perspective. Disabil Rehabil 1996;18:540–549.

24. Lyon JG. Drawing: its value as a communication aid for adults with aphasia. Aphasiology 1995;9:33–94.

25. Garrett KL, Beukelman DR. Severe Aphasia. In KM Yorkston (ed), Augmentative Communication in the Medical Setting. Tucson, AZ: Communication Skill Builders, 1992;245–321.

CHAPTER SEVEN

A Problem-Focused Group Treatment Program for Clients with Mild Aphasia

Robert C. Marshall

In his bestseller, *The Road Less Traveled,* M. Scott Peck says life is difficult because life is full of problems to solve [1]. He also tells us that life would be rather boring without the challenges of problem solving. The neuropsychologist Lezak suggests that problem solving requires conceptualizing, planning, executing, and modifying strategies on the basis of feedback [2]. These skills are compromised by brain injury [3,4], and for some brain-injured persons, this executive function may be impaired independent of successful performance of routine activities [2,5].

This chapter describes a problem-focused group treatment program for clients with mild aphasia at the Veterans Affairs Medical Center, Portland, Oregon. It represents a clinical expansion of earlier reports [6,7] on the use of problem-focused group treatment for clients with mild aphasia. The material herein describes (1) the development and philosophy of the program, (2) participant characteristics, (3) conduct of group sessions and how specific problems were addressed within the group, (4) treatment outcomes, and (5) assessment and documentation strategies.

PROGRAM DEVELOPMENT AND GOALS

System Issues

The Department of Veterans Affairs (VA) is the largest single health care system in the world. This nonprofit 173-hospital system is funded by the U.S. government. It provides a wide range of medical care services (e.g., emergency and acute care, outpatient services, nursing home care) to eligible veterans. VA speech-language pathologists are responsible for assessing and treating communicatively handicapped veterans who have been referred for services. Long-term follow-up of clients who receive speech-language pathology services is facilitated by the reality that veterans who obtain their medical care from the VA rarely leave the system. Because its clients are not charged for services, the number of speech-language pathologists at a particular VA medical center is limited. Staff positions are rarely added if the workload increases because budgets are fixed from year to year and there are no revenues to pay for additional staff. As workload has increased with the aging of the veteran population, VA speech-language pathologists have had to create ways "to do more with less." Because group treatment programs serve more than a single individual, it is not surprising that successful group treatment approaches have been developed in the VA hospitals [6–11].

Circumstantial Issues

In some respects, the motivation for starting the problem-focused group program was circumstantial. For years, I received calls and walk-in visits from clients with mild aphasia who wanted to know how to deal with situations in daily life affected by cognitive-communicative deficits stemming from their aphasia. These clients were beyond the point of needing individualized treatment; however, they intermittently experienced communicative breakdowns secondary to their aphasic deficits that interfered with their ability to solve everyday problems. Typically, the calls and visits took about 30 minutes. I spent this time talking with the client about how to handle his "communication snags," directing him to an appropriate resource, or explaining the nature of the problem he was experiencing. Often, I had to schedule a subsequent 1-hour clinic appointment to cover material that could not be dealt with by phone or in a brief visit. From a practical standpoint, a group situation seemed to be a cost-effective way to handle these types of problems.

Personal Issues

In 1987, I published a paper advocating more services for clients with mild aphasia [12]. I also saw a client who provided the inspiration to start the problem-focused group treatment program. K.L., a 56-year-old man with mild aphasia secondary to a left hemisphere thrombotic stroke, was referred by a private hospital. He was a married, middle-management executive who had tried unsuccessfully to return to work. K.L. was frustrated by this failure; by the incessant demands of his wife and family, who did not see him as impaired, to resume all his pre-stroke responsibilities; and by the slowness with which he performed tasks he had always handled efficiently (e.g., preparing income tax returns, filling out forms). Moreover, he was fearful of having another stroke and worried about finances. For me, K.L. was living proof of Linebaugh's [13] assertion that "the mildness of one's aphasia depends upon the degree to which it impairs the person's ability to communicate at the level demanded by his/her personal, social, vocational, educational, or recreational needs." K.L. and three other men with mild aphasic deficits provided the humble beginnings of the problem-focused group program.

Goals

The primary goal of the problem-focused group program was to give mildly aphasic clients a safe, supportive environment in which to solve problems related to being aphasic. It was hoped that a group situation where clients could receive information and feedback from multiple sources (e.g., group members, facilitator, guest speakers) would be an appropriate vehicle for accomplishing this. More specifically, it was anticipated that a problem-focused group program for clients with mild aphasia would (1) reduce the psychosocial effects of aphasia and improve social, vocational, and recreational integration [14]; (2) give clients information to enable them to discuss the physical, psychological, and social consequences of brain injury; and (3) give clients space to develop initiative [15].

PARTICIPANT CHARACTERISTICS

Criteria for group membership were not developed a priori. Certain characteristics, however, distinguished participants in this group from other aphasic people. In addition, it became apparent that not all mildly aphasic clients were candidates for the problem-focused group, and some who at first appeared to be good candidates were not able to participate in the group. This awareness guided decisions about who should and should not participate in the group.

Characteristics of Group Members

Independence
Aphasic clients have been described on a continuum of cognitive-communicative independence [7]. Dependent clients have severe speech, language, cognitive, and physical deficits. Their self-care needs may preclude living at home, and many are residents of long-term care facilities. They depend on their significant others or caregivers for meeting their basic needs. In contrast, all participants in this program lived at home, either alone, with a significant other, or with a family member. All were capable of getting to and from scheduled group sessions independently (driving, walking, using public transportation). All had "functional communication." Although these independent clients had less severe cognitive-communicative deficits, their language abilities were susceptible to breakdown under stress, time pressure, and fatigue. Some had withdrawn from social, vocational, recreational, and other situations that demanded communication and were frustrated by their aphasic deficits.

Speech and Language Skills
Previous reports of clients in problem-focused groups have shown that their scores on standardized tests are often within normal limits [6]. My program used discussion as the primary vehicle for solving problems. Traditional foci of aphasia treatment (e.g., word retrieval skills, sentence expansion) received limited consideration. Group members needed to be able to ask questions and initiate topics for discussion. Clients with motor speech problems, such as dysarthria and apraxia of speech, often had difficulty keeping up with group discussions. Clients with severe word-finding problems or long response latencies exhibited similar problems. Standardized tests, such as the Porch Index of Communicative Ability (PICA) [16] and Boston Naming Test (BNT) [17] were not always good predictors of a client's ability to participate in the group. For example, some fluent clients were fully capable of participating in group discussions despite relatively low scores on measures such as the PICA and BNT. More often, speed, fluency, and persistence not to compromise the integrity of messages were better predictors of group participation than scores from standardized tests of verbal function.

Medical Status
Clients undergoing treatment of medical problems secondary to a stroke (e.g., with frequent visits to the doctor, medication adjustments, laboratory studies) tended to have different needs and concerns than those who were further post-onset and medically stable. For this reason, clients were seldom started in the problem-focused group until 3 months post-onset and after they had been living at home for a while.

Group Membership

Attendance
Often, issues of concern for group members could not be completely resolved in a single session. It became apparent that regular attendance by group members was needed to ensure continuity of the discussions from session to session. One factor affecting attendance was whether the group member assumed responsibility for getting to and from the session. When a group member needed to depend on another person for transportation to and from the group meeting, attendance was sporadic. Therefore, availability and ease of transportation became a "soft" selection criterion for admitting a client to the group.

Pragmatic Skills
Some clients did not have the interpersonal skills to participate in a group. For example, client C.T. joined the group after a left hemisphere stroke with resulting mild right hemiparesis and mild aphasia. C.T.'s primary concern was himself. His typical behavioral pattern was (1) to come to the first half of the group meeting, (2) to ask his specific questions (e.g., "Who do I talk to about getting a bus pass?"), and (3) after obtaining this information, to leave the meeting abruptly. Inability or unwillingness to listen was another deterrent to group participation. Client C.K. participated avidly as long as the discussion was related to his particular concerns, but he "clammed up" when the discussion centered on another group member. Hypercritical individuals also tended to make poor group members. Client L.P. tended to roll his eyes and make disparaging comments when another group member brought up a topic that he thought was silly. Because group participation required a certain degree of pragmatic competence, group members were allowed to provide input on whether a new client should join the group. This decision usually came after the prospective group member had attended three or four group meetings on a trial basis.

Age
Some differences were related to the age of group participants. At the initial stages of the program, group participants tended to be older, retired, have grown children, and be in long-term marriages. Younger clients were often working when they became aphasic; some had children at home; some were married, and some were not. Their concerns centered on relationships, child rearing, work, and

finances, whereas older group participants tended to be more concerned with leisure activities (e.g., travel, playing cards), medical issues, and decision making (e.g., "Should I paint my house?"). Over time, it became necessary to have separate groups for older and younger clients.

GROUP STRUCTURE

Problem-focused groups met once per week for 60–90 minutes. As group facilitator, the clinician attempted to focus and clarify discussion topics, ensure equitable participation, record the proceedings, and, when necessary, review material that had not been processed in prior sessions. Group members were responsible for identifying specific problems and working together toward solutions. Solutions to problems and tactics for dealing with specific situations were facilitated by tapping the expertise and knowledge of group members with diverse backgrounds and experiences. Typically, when one client identified a problem, another client had encountered the same problem or had the requisite background (e.g., as a physician or attorney) to offer some suggestions for managing the problem. Treatment specifics are best understood with some concrete examples. Some of the following examples reflect problem-solving activities involving the entire group. Others reflect problems brought up by individual group members that were solved in the group setting.

Examples of Group Problem Solving

Compensating for Slowed Processing
Although mildly aphasic clients can perform many pre-stroke tasks, it often takes them longer to complete the tasks. When they try to speed up, they tend to make more mistakes and become frustrated. Clients K.D. and C.L. complained about how long it took them to assemble a furnace and a barbecue. Client J.F. was frustrated with the time it took him to perform routine maintenance on his car. Some plausible options discussed in the group were to (1) lay out the tools and parts needed for the task in their proper order before starting the task; (2) allow enough time to accomplish the task; (3) schedule the task at a time, preferably the morning, when the client was functioning optimally; and (4) check the accuracy of his work step by step.

Preparedness
Mildly aphasic clients need to prepare themselves for situations in which their language processing skills will be taxed. Preparedness relates to Eisenson's suggestion that high-level aphasic clients do what they can to avoid making quick statements and snap judgments and to establish reputations as "deep thinkers" [18]. This was seen with client C.C., who agonized over having to write a check at the market when there were people in line behind her. It was suggested that she write the check before getting to the cashier's stand and ask the clerk to fill in the proper

amount. Similarly, client S.P. was worried about an impending appointment with his physician because the physician had moved his office to a new location. He feared getting lost, being late, and having to ask for directions. Solutions proposed were to (1) look at a city map and (2) make a trial run to the new location a day or two ahead of time to become familiar with the route.

Communicating in an Emergency
An oft-cited fear of clients with brain injury is that they will encounter an emergency situation in which they need to communicate effectively but cannot do so [6]. Clients might think that they will be perceived as drunk or mentally incompetent. In one group session, individual identification cards were made to use in emergency situations in which communication problems secondary to aphasia were anticipated. These cards provide several functions: (1) informing the reader that the client is an aphasic stroke victim who has problems speaking in pressured situations and that the client has no difficulty understanding; (2) stipulating how to speak with the client; and (3) designating who to call for help.

Doctor's Appointment
Some clients became anxious about doctor's appointments. Concerns were not having enough time to ask questions about their health or not being able to remember what the physician told them. The group identified ways to handle this predicament: (1) rehearse or write down important questions before the appointment, and (2) ask the physician to write down any recommendations provided. Clients were further advised to procure information pamphlets on their particular medical conditions (e.g., diabetes) and general health issues (e.g., effects of smoking), to review this information, and, if it was felt to be helpful, to use it to formulate their questions. Client M.W. suggested that information advice lines were commonplace in most medical facilities and that he had benefited from using them.

Self-Disclosure
Mildly aphasic clients struggle with when and if to tell a listener that they had had a stroke and may have difficulty communicating in certain situations. They discussed occasions where it might be appropriate and advantageous to inform a listener about the stroke and resulting aphasia, as well as occasions when this information should not be disclosed. Clients shared experiences about when it was helpful to disarm their listener with a statement such as, "Two years ago I had a stroke and sometimes it affects my speech." For example, client L.B. said that he received more prompt, courteous service when purchasing tires after he told the salesman about his stroke. Another client reported that he was given more time to complete his messages if he informed his listeners that he had had a stroke.

Anger
Mildly aphasic clients often express dissatisfaction with listeners' intolerance for their communicative deficits. Like

all people, they like to be treated respectfully. Frequently, it was necessary to spend some time discussing how a client might have dealt with an unpleasant situation or how she would handle a future situation if she felt she had been treated rudely. For example, client S.B. needed to purchase parts for his car. S.B. had three specific items clearly in mind when he approached the service counter. Unfortunately, he also had a severe word retrieval block when the clerk said, "May I help you?" Initially, S.B. stalled for time by describing the mechanical problem with his car. The clerk then tried to supply the missing words by guessing, but this only caused S.B. to get more frustrated. Ultimately, S.B. said "Forget it" and left the store. S.B. felt that he had had "the last word," but group members pointed out that his reaction undermined his goal (to get the parts for his car). It was suggested that in the future, S.B. make a list of the items he needed before going to the store. A discussion about responsibility and communicative burden followed. Eventually, most clients agreed with Eisenson's belief that aphasic people need to realize that it is not the listener's task to figure out the gist of the message or to divine the aphasic speaker's mood and intent [18]. Specific behavioral tactics were proposed: keeping calm, walking away from situations gracefully, and, when necessary, taking a break from the action to minimize angry feelings.

Individual Problem-Solving Examples

Usually, the session time was spent solving problems that were unique to individual group members. The following sections detail examples of individual concerns that were resolved within the problem-focused group.

Child Custody

Client J.B. was a 42-year-old man whose left hemisphere embolic stroke involving the temporal-parietal area resulted in a fluent aphasia. His former wife felt that his stroke warranted her having complete custody of their 12-year-old son. J.B. seemed to be capable of caring for his son despite his aphasic deficits. His ability to run the household, shop, cook, manage finances, and monitor his son's school work did not change as a result of his stroke. Moreover, J.B. adequately communicated with his son, and his son, on observation, had no difficulty communicating with J.B. Unfortunately, J.B. and his ex-wife communicated only via their attorneys. The group came up with an excellent suggestion: to have J.B. evaluated by a behavioral neurologist, who would then write a letter documenting his competency as a single parent. This strategy worked perfectly, and the custody issue was resolved without delay.

Managing Finances

S.D. was a 70-year-old widow with chronic aphasia secondary to a thromboembolic stroke. She lived in her own home and supported herself on a pension. In what she described as "a weak moment," she loaned a sum of money to her 42-year-old unemployed daughter. The daughter promised to repay the loan promptly but did not do so. S.D. came to a group meeting "seething" over the circumstance. The immediate problem was that S.D. was so angry over her daughter's treatment that she was no longer communicating effectively. She rejected all suggestions to recover the funds legally. The eventual outcome, albeit not a happy one for S.D., was that "we all need to learn from our mistakes." After a group discussion, S.D. agreed to forgive the bad debt and vowed to be cautious in loaning her daughter money in the future. On another occasion, S.D. signed up for a credit card through a mail offer. Thrilled with the low monthly payments, she made several purchases. To her surprise, she learned that the interest charged for credit on her purchases exceeded her monthly income. This time her reactions were more intense. She became so upset she could not sleep. She started taking tranquilizers to such an extent that her physician became concerned and diagnosed her as depressed. S.D. considered declaring bankruptcy. Members of the group with business experience explained the concept of interest to S.D. They also explained the disadvantages associated with bankruptcy. The final solution to this problem was for S.D. to work with a consumer credit counselor, set up a plan for paying her bills, and re-establish financial solvency.

Employment

Although returning to work after a stroke can be problematic, some mildly aphasic clients do not want to stop working. Too often, physicians equate stroke with disability retirement. This happened to client J.H., a 63-year-old man who had a left hemisphere stroke that minimally affected his speech but left him with no physical impairments. The attending physician felt that J.H. would need to retire. He did not know, however, that J.H.'s job as a file clerk placed few demands on his communication skills. In the group, J.H. explained the nature of his job and that 2 more years of work on the job would give him a much-needed pension. Group members encouraged him not to retire. It was suggested that the speech-language pathologist call the employer and determine the communicative demands of the job, and that J.H. return to work part time. J.H. did that, and in 2 weeks he was able to resume full-time employment.

Another client, E.H., expressed problems making ends meet on his meager pension. He wanted to earn a supplementary income. This 56-year-old man with moderately severe Broca's aphasia could not handle a job with communicative demands, but he did feel he could work as a part-time janitor. Interviewing for a job was problematic because of his aphasia. Possible vocational counseling was discussed. The group drafted a letter detailing E.H.'s assets (e.g., dependability, physical ability to do the janitorial work) and liabilities (communicating). Eventually the clinician wrote such a letter. Ultimately, E.H. was hired as a nighttime janitor and was able to supplement his income significantly. This allowed him to work without worrying about communicative demands.

With respect to clients' feelings about work, it is commonplace to hear comments such as "I used to be an attorney," "I used to make $40,000 per year," and "I was considered one of the best mechanics in the area." When clients perceive that a new job represents a step backward, they can become discouraged. This happened with client K.L., who, like E.H., also needed to earn extra money. As mentioned earlier, K.L. had tried without success to return to his former job. He also tried unsuccessfully to start a similar business on his own. He had many talents, however: He was a master gardener and was physically fit. With some encouragement from the group and constant reminding that the goal was to augment his income, not regain his former status, he started a landscaping business and assumed a paper route.

Negotiating the Bureaucracy

When the aphasic client is working at the time of a stroke, he becomes a candidate for Social Security Disability (SSD). If the employer is providing health insurance when the stroke occurs, this coverage is often discontinued, and the individual is converted to Medicare in approximately 2 years. These supplementary insurance benefits are often the primary support for aphasic stroke victims. The phrase *negotiating the bureaucracy* refers to all the red tape a brain-injured person must go through to obtain these benefits. Some, but not all, of these steps include (1) making appointments, (2) obtaining proper forms, (3) filling out the forms, (4) being interviewed by phone, (5) obtaining copies of medical records, and (6) being examined by physicians and neuropsychologists. Completion of these tasks taps cognitive-communicative skills at the highest level. Obtaining the much-needed SSD is complicated by two issues. First, for many mildly aphasic persons, brain injury is invisible: The client has functional communication and no obvious physical deficits, yet still cannot be gainfully employed. Second, most clients and their families are confused by the myriad forms required by the system and do not seek assistance in completing them. Their attitude is expressed by "I have suffered a stroke. I cannot work, and therefore I will receive disability." Their response when they are denied SSD, as is so often the case on the first application, can be catastrophic.

After wading through the morass of forms, appointments, and requirements to qualify for SSD, clients learn how the system works. Members of the group were more than willing to share their personal experiences in negotiating the bureaucracy. Collectively, the group's knowledge of this subject was awesome. This expertise was often put to good use with new group members and clients who had failed to obtain SSD with their first application. In most instances, someone knew (1) where and who to call, (2) what and how to write, (3) who to see for an examination, and (4) proper and improper ways to complete forms. When a client learns how to navigate one bureaucratic system, he learns skills that often facilitate moving through other systems. Some of these skills include (1) obtaining low-cost government-sponsored housing, (2) qualifying for real estate tax reductions, (3) procuring senior citizen bus passes, (4) obtaining free or reduced-rate fishing and hunting licenses, (5) obtaining specific veteran benefits, and (6) finding out about low-cost or free meal programs. The communicative demands required for these activities are challenging, varying, and personally relevant. They provide fantastic therapy material.

Social Contacts

The final example is a group problem-solving effort that led to a very positive personal experience for the clinician. Client L.P., a widower, was lonely but feared dating because his word-finding difficulties were embarrassing. A social worker from the organization Adults Without Partners was invited to talk to the group about meeting new people. The group suggested that L.P. write a personal advertisement about himself for a local paper. The details of the advertisement were discussed in group meetings. After he received many responses to the advertisement, more problem-focused discussion ensued: Which responses would be answered? Should he inform the woman that he had had a stroke? Should this be done before or after the first meeting? Should he respond by phone or in writing? L.P.'s success stimulated the clinician to create an advertisement. Ultimately, L.P. and the clinician both met and eventually married respondents to their respective advertisements.

OUTCOMES

Several writers have stressed that the use of group therapy must be supported by empiric data [19–21]. Traditionally, these data have come in the form of pre- and post-treatment comparisons that show the client has improved in some measurable way on a standardized test [8,9,11,22]. Mildly aphasic clients, however, have little room for improvement on these tests [6,23].

The most valuable overall outcome of problem-focused group therapy is that it stimulates increased participation in life for its members. Some aphasia literature has suggested that this factor can reduce handicaps and may actually be a more preferred goal of aphasia treatment than improving speech, given the lack of generalization of traditional aphasia treatment in natural settings [24–26]. Three generally beneficial outcomes appear to be associated with the problem-focused group treatment: (1) the solving of problems of immediate concern to a client, thereby enabling him or her to move ahead in life; (2) increased opportunities for socialization; and (3) support.

Problem Solving

Several examples of how specific problems were addressed in the group situation have been provided. It is difficult to estimate the value of solving a specific problem for the individual, however, or to specify how this might benefit the health care system. Consider the case of client S.D., who was abusing tranquilizers because she was depressed about her credit card debt. Did the intervention reduce the number of contacts S.D. had with her physician? Did it prevent further abuse, subsequent illness, and perhaps keep her from having to move from an independent to an assisted living situation? What are the benefits of J.H.'s returning to work? Does society benefit from the taxes he pays on this income, his health insurance coverage continuing at the employer's expense, and the fact that he will not apply for SSD? What is the value of a client being able to resume an activity (e.g., playing poker with friends) that was abandoned after a stroke? We do not know the answers to any of these questions, and we will not find them in traditional paradigms. Significantly, Lyon and colleagues [25] found that aphasic adults who participated in a program designed to enhance participation in life in natural settings improved on two measures of well-being and communication constructed by the investigators but not on other measures.

Socialization

For most clients, the group was an important social event of the week. The scheduled meeting provided opportunities for members to meet and to discuss current events before the session, have lunch afterward, and plan activities of mutual interest (e.g., camping, hot-tubbing, fishing, shopping for a car). Some group members hosted potlucks, picnics, and barbecues at their homes, inviting group members and their families. The problem-focused group tended to attract mildly aphasic people who had been "doers" rather than passive participants. Most clients wanted to continue or to resume participation in their pre-stroke activities but showed reduced initiative. There may indeed be safety in numbers and in knowing that others have similar problems with initiative. These factors may have provided the impetus for participants to resume social activities that they had enjoyed before the stroke.

Support

Support refers to educating aphasic clients and their families about the nature of aphasia and its impact on the family [27]. Sources of support can be personal (e.g., friends and family), community (e.g., stroke clubs), and professional. The nature of the support received can be emotional and informational [28]. Members of the problem-focused group functioned as a social support system for each other. Cantor [29] defines a social support system as "a pattern of continuous or intermittent ties and interchanges of mutual assistance that plays a significant role in maintaining the psychological, social, and physical integrity of the individual over time." One of the most vivid examples of the group serving as a support system occurred when a group member and his wife were legally separated. This client had a limited income, no household supplies, and no means of transportation. Group members went to their garages, their attics, and garage sales to put together the items he needed to furnish his apartment.

ASSESSMENT AND DOCUMENTATION

Assessment

Most participants in the problem-focused group had received individual treatment before entering the group. All had been thoroughly assessed with a variety of instruments before starting the group. Unfortunately, measures such as the BNT, PICA, Token Test [30], and other traditional tests are insensitive to long-term changes in functional communication performance of people with mild aphasia [6,23,31]. Moreover, many of the changes seen in group members reflected increased participation in life activities and a reduction in their handicap.

Documentation

It was necessary to document the progress of individual group members. It was helpful to do this at longer intervals than usual (e.g., every 6 months rather than every month) because of the chronic nature of clients' mild aphasia. The following sections describe some of the documentation methods used.

Standardized Tests
In a previous paper of mine [6], the problem-focused group treatment program reflected slight pre- and posttest improvements on the PICA after group therapy for 14 of 18 patients. Standardized tests are most useful within the first year after a stroke that results in aphasia. Longterm changes are more appropriately documented in other ways.

Client Self-Reports
Verbal client self-reports to persons unfamiliar with aphasia provide useful information about how the client functions outside the group. One way of doing this was to have a first-year graduate student in speech-language pathology conduct an unstructured interview with the client to determine the client's level of participation in communicative activities of daily living. Comparative interviews from year to year often illustrate that the client is more actively involved in activities from one year to the next.

Exit Interviews
It was sometimes useful to ask clients who were leaving the group what they felt they accomplished as a result of being a group member. Exit interviews were unstructured and usually began with the request, "Tell me how you think this group has helped." This information was videotaped to provide a permanent record of how the client felt treatment had helped him or her.

Communicative Effectiveness Index
The Communicative Effectiveness Index [32] can be used to document changes in people who are mildly aphasic. With this instrument, the client, significant other, or clinician rates 16 items (e.g., starting up a conversation with people who are not close family) by plac-

ing a mark on a 10-cm visual analog scale. The scale's anchor points are "Not at all able" or "As well as before the stroke." Ratings are averaged to provide an overall index, and the difference in overall ratings from one assessment to the next provides a measure of improvement. The American Speech-Hearing-Language Association Functional Assessment of Communication Skills for Adults also appears to be a viable measure for documenting individual change secondary to treatment in the problem-focused group [33].

Problem-Solving Inventory

The Problem-Solving Inventory (PSI) is a set of scales that estimate the individual's ability to solve real-life problems [34]. The purpose of the PSI is to assess an individual's perceptions of his own problem-solving behaviors and attitudes. This 35-item instrument consists of three scales: problem-solving confidence, approach-avoidance style, and personal control. The total PSI score is a general index of problem-solving abilities.

Group Progress Notes

Progress notes were written monthly in the client's medical chart. These notes began with a boilerplate statement about the purpose of the group, the client's attendance record, and specific issues the client addressed in the past month. Progress notes identified behaviors, such as risk taking and evaluative thinking, that reflected the benefits of problem-focused group treatment. Risk taking involves attempting an activity or task that the client had given up after the stroke or starting a new activity. Evaluative thinking involves obtaining relevant information about a problem [35] and arriving independently at the best decision. For example, one client obtained contractors' bids on painting her house and made a decision about the project. The year before she had not been able to make this decision.

Discharge and Reimbursement Issues

Clients were allowed to attend the group as long as they wished. Some clients discharged themselves; others became too ill to participate. Clients were not charged for attending the group. The estimate of what it cost to run the group was approximately $5 per session per person. This figure was derived by dividing the clinician's salary, fringe benefits, and other overhead costs by the number of persons attending the group (usually eight to 10).

CONCLUSION

The clinician's experience with the program was that it helped a lot of mildly aphasic people lead more enjoyable, productive lives. Mild aphasic deficits, as demonstrated by clients in this group, constitute a handicap, as defined by the World Health Organization (WHO) [36]. In WHO terminology, a handicap results when discor-

dance occurs between the person's performance or status and the expectations of the societal group to which the person belongs. For some mildly aphasic persons [12], aphasia is no less handicapping than it is for a severely aphasic person. Because most mildly aphasic clients have re-established functional communication when they are referred to the speech-language pathologist, the ways in which their aphasic deficits impair participation in life may be overlooked. Accordingly, some writers have suggested that our concept of functional communication warrants expansion [24,37]. The problem-focused group approach offers a potential avenue for addressing the problems of aphasic people who may "fall through the cracks" of the rehabilitation system because they have functional communication at the time of referral and are erroneously seen as not in need of treatment. In a frequently cited chapter on group therapy, Kearns [21] considers the problem-focused group a multipurpose cohort that provides a forum for discussing social, vocational, and recreational reintegration into society and assisting clients in solving everyday communication problems. It is hoped that the foregoing examples prove his appraisal accurate.

Acknowledgements

The author gratefully acknowledges the guidance, good will, and cooperation of clients who formed the nucleus of the problem-focused group and all the aphasic clients who participated, including John D., Bob C., Bob J., Norm R., George J., Cecile M., Ben H., Ralph W., Bill W., Jim M., Pat N., Mike P., Tom M., Carol M., Dick B., Hal B., Jeri B., Ed B., and Gerry B. It was a pleasure and a privilege to facilitate this group. The author is also indebted to Claudia A. Morelli for her careful editing and assistance with this manuscript.

REFERENCES

1. Peck S. The Road Less Traveled. New York: Simon & Schuster, 1973;3–4.
2. Lezak M. Neuropsychological Assessment (2nd ed). New York: Oxford University Press, 1983.
3. Glosser G, Goodglass H. Disorders of executive control functions among aphasic and other brain damaged patients. J Clin Exp Psych 1990;12:485–501.
4. Ben-Yishay Y, Diller L. Cognitive Remediation. In M Rosenthal, E Griffith, M Bond, R Miller (eds), Remediation of the Head Injured Adult. Philadelphia: Davis, 1983;76–95.
5. Vilkki J. Problem-solving deficits after focal cerebral lesions. Cortex 1988;24:119–127.
6. Marshall RC. Problem-focused group treatment for clients with mild aphasia. Am J Speech Lang Pathol 1993;2:31–37.
7. Marshall RC. Falling through the cracks: the dilemma of mild aphasia. Presented at the American Speech-Hearing-Language Association Convention, Anaheim, CA, 1993.
8. Aten J, Caliguri M, Holland A. The efficacy of functional communication therapy for chronic aphasic patients. J Speech Hear Disord 1982;47:559–561.
9. Bollinger R, Musson N, Holland A. A study of group communication intervention with chronically aphasic persons. Aphasiology 1993;7:301–313.
10. Kearns K, Simmons N. Group therapy for aphasia: a survey of V.A. medical centers. Clin Aphasiol 1985;15:176–183.

11. Wertz RT, Collins M, Weiss D, et al. Veterans Administration cooperative study on aphasia: a comparison of individual and group treatment. J Speech Hear Disord 1981;24:580–594.
12. Marshall RC. Reapportioning time for aphasia rehabilitation: a point of view. Aphasiology 1987;1:59–74.
13. Linebaugh C. Mild Aphasia. In A Holland (ed), Language Disorders in Adults. San Diego: College Hill, 1984;113–132.
14. Springer L. Facilitating group rehabilitation. Aphasiology 1991;5:563–565.
15. Repo M. The holistic approach to rehabilitation. Aphasiology 1991;5:571–572.
16. Porch BE. Porch Index of Communicative Ability. Palo Alto, CA: Consulting Psychologists, 1981.
17. Kaplan E, Goodglass H, Weintraub S. Boston Naming Test. Philadelphia: Lea & Febiger, 1983.
18. Eisenson J. The Recovered Aphasic: Residual Problems and Vocational Implications. In J Eisenson (ed), Adult Aphasia. New York: Appleton-Century-Crofts, 1973;192–203.
19. Aten J. Group therapy for aphasic patients: let's show it works. Aphasiology 1991;5:559–561.
20. Fawcus M. Group Therapy: A Learning Situation. In C Code, D Muller (eds), Aphasia Therapy (2nd ed). London: Cole & Whurr, 1989;113–119.
21. Kearns K. Group Therapy for Aphasia: Theoretical and Practical Considerations. In R Chapey (ed), Language Intervention Strategies in Adult Aphasia (3rd ed). Baltimore: Williams & Wilkins, 1994;304–321.
22. Elman R, Bernstein-Ellis E. Effectiveness of group communication treatment for individuals with chronic aphasia: results of communicative and linguistic measures. Presented at the Clinical Aphasiology Conference, Newport, RI, 1996.
23. Raymer A, LaPointe LL. The nature and assessment of the mildly impaired aphasic person. Semin Speech Lang 1986;7:207–220.
24. Lyon J. Communication use and participation in life for adults with aphasia in natural settings: the scope of the problem. Am J Speech Lang Pathol 1992;1:7–14.
25. Lyon J, Cariski D, Keisler L, et al. Communication partners: enhancing participation in life and communication for adults with aphasia in natural settings. Aphasiology 1997;11:667–679.
26. Kagan A, Gailey L. Functional Is Not Enough: Training Conversation Partners for Aphasic Adults. In A Holland, M Forbes (eds), Aphasia Treatment: World Perspectives. London: Chapman & Hall, 1993;199–226.
27. Brookshire R. An Introduction to Aphasia and Related Disorders. St Louis: Mosby–Year Book, 1992.
28. Friedland J, McColl M. Social support for stroke survivors: development and evaluation of an intervention program. Phys Occ Ther Geriat 1989;7:55–69.
29. Cantor M. The Informal Support System: Its Relationship in the Lives of the Elderly. In E Borgotta, N McClusky (eds), Aging and Society. Beverly Hills, CA: Sage Publications, 1980;131–144.
30. DeRenzi E, Vignolo L. The Token Test: a sensitive test to detect receptive disturbances in aphasics. Brain 1962;85:665–678.
31. Darley FL. Aphasia. Philadelphia: Saunders, 1982.
32. Lomas J, Pikard L, Bester S, et al. The Communicative Effectiveness Index: development and psychometric evaluation of a functional communication measure for adult aphasia. J Speech Hear Disord 1989;54:113–123.
33. Fratteli C, Thompson C, Holland A, et al. Functional Assessment of Communication Skills for Adults. Rockville, MD: American Speech-Language-Hearing Association, 1996.
34. Heppner PP. The Problem Solving Inventory. Palo Alto, CA: Consulting Psychologists, 1988.
35. Chapey R. Cognitive Intervention: Stimulation of Cognition, Memory, Convergent Thinking, Divergent Thinking and Evaluative Thinking. In R Chapey (ed), Language Intervention Strategies in Adult Aphasia. Baltimore: Williams & Wilkins, 1994;220–245.
36. World Health Organization. International Classification of Impairments, Disabilities, and Handicaps. Geneva, Switzerland: WHO, 1980.
37. Elman R, Bernstein-Ellis E. What is functional? Am J Speech Lang Pathol 1995;4:115–117.

Part Two: University and Student-Facilitated Groups

CHAPTER EIGHT

An Alternative Model for the Treatment of Aphasia: The LifeLink© Approach

Delaina Walker-Batson,
Sandra Curtis, Patricia Smith,
and Jean Ford

The challenge health care professionals face is to develop alternative delivery models that extend opportunities for rehabilitation to patients in the chronic phases of recovery. It is not feasible to expect optimal patient outcomes, given the limited number of visits for rehabilitation funded in today's health care market. The Texas Woman's University Aphasia Center–Dallas is a successful alternative transdisciplinary environment for graduate students in training, volunteers, and certified professionals to provide services to individuals with aphasia. The Aphasia Center operates 2½ days per week. Two days are for individual and group treatment, and the half day is for LifeLink© activities. The program has three levels of delivery, which depend on the communication ability and functional independence of the client. This model can easily be implemented in other academic settings that train allied health professionals. Parts of the model are applicable to more traditional delivery environments.

PHILOSOPHY OF PROGRAM

The philosophy underlying our approach is both holistic and ecologic. Each individual with aphasia interacts in a complex, interdependent system. We believe that the treatment of aphasia must look at the whole person and the interaction of that whole person with his or her unique environment. This holistic approach acknowledges the importance of psychosocial factors (besides communication) in the recovery process and targets quality of life and client and caregiver perceptions of well-being as viable outcome measures [1]. The model that we use is ecologic [2–5] in that we believe that generalization must be planned, orchestrated, and implemented for carryover into daily life. Although ecologic in philosophy, our approach does not eliminate traditional principles of applied behavioral science. Research in recovery of function after brain injury provides strong evidence that for neurologic as well as behavioral change to occur, there must be much redundancy with practice in specifically targeted behaviors [6]. Our approach is a hybrid of traditional and functional treatment.

LifeLink©

The basis of our model is a concept called LifeLink©, which provides a bridge to what we believe should be the primary outcome of treatment—participation in life. Through LifeLink©, we plan theme-based activities that systematically prepare clients for community re-entry, beginning with individual treatment and continuing into community outings. Participation in planned everyday life activities often results in changes in the client's perception of self and psychosocial well-being.

The LifeLink© Program

The LifeLink© program is an activity-based, half-day program. Activities may be an extension of a specifically developed theme (e.g., bird watching, art lessons, meal preparation), a social activity (e.g., a holiday luncheon), or an exploration of community resources (e.g., attending a sporting event, riding mass transit). These activities give clients social opportunities in which to practice communication skills and build confidence in their ability to participate fully in life. A key component of the LifeLink© program is the development of avocational and leisure interests.

Transdisciplinary Environment

The transdisciplinary environment at the Aphasia Center complements the focused aphasia program and enhances community independence. A transdisciplinary approach to care includes the client and his or her primary support system as essential members of the rehabilitation team. The health care professionals on the team are those with essential skills to facilitate the rehabilitation process for a specific diagnosis. Speech-language pathology, physical therapy, occupational therapy, nursing, and social work are represented on the team at the Aphasia Center. Each professional on the team performs discipline-specific assessments. Program planning is based on the results of the assessments in conjunction with the client's past medical and social history as well as his or her present functional needs and preferences. Treatment tasks for the client can be categorized as those that are novel or familiar. Novel tasks require treatment by the professional as new skills are learned. Once the task is familiar, other professionals and family members can practice it. This concept of shared practice affords the client many opportunities to practice tasks, with the goal of becoming skilled enough at the tasks to be able to generalize the tasks to any environment.

Ecologic Nature of Treatment

We use environmentally relevant themes to pair traditional and functional treatment. Themes or topics provide the content for therapy sessions and determine the therapy contexts of simulated and real-life experiences. We have found that themes are an excellent vehicle for providing continuity, cohesiveness, and redundancy that can be applied in all modalities. A thematically related, large, core vocabulary is established, which makes it more likely that generalization will occur. Themes can be recycled as recovery occurs, with an expansion in core vocabulary and an increase in task demands. The transdisciplinary approach is enhanced when all team members are focused on a theme and related outcomes. Themes serve two purposes that are not mutually exclusive. Some themes are developed by the transdisciplinary team to focus on functional outcomes to facilitate the client reclaiming or redefining roles in the home and the community. The focus of other themes is for enhancing communicative competence and developing leisure activities.

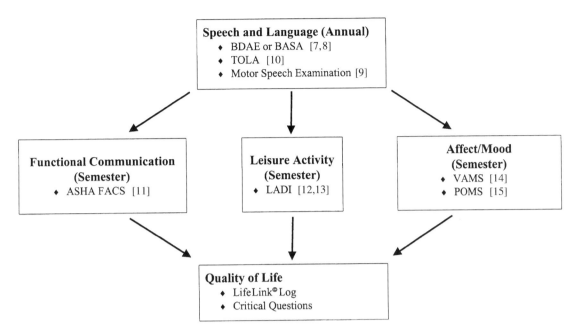

FIGURE 8-1.   The Aphasia Center assessment schedule. (BDAE = Boston Diagnostic Aphasia Examination; BASA = Boston Assessment of Severe Aphasia; TOLA = Test of Oral and Limb Apraxia; ASHA FACS = American Speech-Language-Hearing Association Functional Assessment of Communication Skills for Adults; LADI = Leisure Activity Development Index; VAMS = Visual Analogue Mood Scale; POMS = Profile of Mood States.)

Psychosocial Support Groups

The Aphasia Center provides weekly psychosocial support groups for clients and family members to promote psychosocial well-being. Membership in the client group is limited to individuals who can benefit from a group problem-solving process. The family support group is open to all family members. The social worker meets with family members to discuss issues and problems and provide support. The psychiatric nurse helps the client group to work through problems that the clients have identified. The co-facilitator of this group is a client who has aphasia and experience with group process. To maintain confidentiality, other professionals on the transdisciplinary team, volunteers, and students do not participate in this group.

Graduate Student Training

The Aphasia Center is a demonstration and training center for graduate students in speech-language pathology, physical therapy, and occupational therapy. Approximately 10 students from each discipline are assigned every semester to serve 30 clients with aphasia. Students in all disciplines are required to complete a basic neurology course before a practicum assignment at the center. Most students have had no prior experience with stroke and aphasia. A transdisciplinary orientation by professional staff in all disciplines, held at the beginning of each semester, addresses such things as clinical procedures, therapeutic techniques, and shared practice opportunities. Weekly staff meetings are held for transdisciplinary client management and direct clinical application of principles and theories from academic courses.

ENTRY CRITERIA

Clients who participate in the Aphasia Center must have had a left hemisphere brain injury resulting in aphasia, be at least 18 years of age, and be independent in toileting (or have a caregiver on-site). After referral, a pre-intake screening interview with the client and significant other is scheduled with the center's director. If it is determined that the Aphasia Center is the appropriate setting for the client, a complete diagnostic assessment is scheduled.

ASSESSMENT AND DOCUMENTATION OF PROGRESS

A holistic assessment of each client includes assessment of speech and language abilities, functional communication, leisure activity participation, mood, and affect. Figure 8-1 shows each domain, the names of assessment tools, and frequency of administration. After admission to the center, the patient undergoes assessments by physical therapy and occupational therapy. These assessments review motor and sensory impairments and the impact of the impairments on functional task performance. The psychiatric nurse assesses clients who participate in the psychosocial support group for depression. Figure 8-2 lists the transdisciplinary assessments.

Physical Therapy

♦ Fugl-Meyer Motor Scale [22]
♦ Mathias Get Up & Go [23]
♦ Barthel [24]

Occupational Therapy

♦ Canadian Occupational
  Performance Measure [25]

Psychiatric Nursing

♦ Geriatric Screening
  Depression Scale [26]

FIGURE 8-2.   **Transdisciplinary assessments.**

Speech and Language Assessments

The Boston Diagnostic Aphasia Examination (BDAE) [7] or the Boston Assessment of Severe Aphasia [8] is administered to sample speech and language behavior in all modalities (auditory comprehension, verbal expression, reading and writing), to determine the severity of aphasia, and to provide information for the focus of treatment activities. Short forms of the Mayo Clinic Motor Speech Assessment [9] and the Test of Oral and Limb Apraxia [10] are administered if indicated. Informal assessment of communicative success and efficiency in use of alternative communication, such as drawing, gesturing, or communication notebook use, is conducted if appropriate. Functional communication is assessed both formally and informally. The American Speech-Language-Hearing Association Functional Assessment of Communication Skills for Adults [11] is the primary functional assessment tool used to measure social communication; basic needs; reading, writing, and number concepts; and daily planning ability. In addition, family interaction is observed to determine (1) if the established system of communication is adaptive or maladaptive, (2) who carries the burden of communication, (3) strategies used by the client, and (4) facilitative communication strategies used by communication partners.

Leisure Activity Assessment

As an index of psychosocial adjustment, we have modified an approach used in occupational therapy [12] to deter-

mine the number of hours per week each client spends in leisure activities. This assessment, the Leisure Activity Development Index, was developed and pilot tested for use at the center [13]. It is used to determine if the client is taking a passive or active role in leisure activity and to what extent he or she participates in eight categories of leisure activity.

Mood and Affect Assessment

The Visual Analogue Mood Scale [14] and the Profile of Mood States [15] are used to assess mood and affect. Because of the complexity of assessing affect and mood in individuals with varying degrees of aphasia, numerous scales of affect and mood were field tested [16], and these two measures were determined, with some modifications, to have the greatest usability.

Quality of Life Assessment

Assessment of quality of life is done primarily through the LifeLink© Log and a structured interview of six critical questions [4]. These assessments document changes in the client's perception of self, autonomy, positive relationships with others, personal growth, mastery of environment, and life goals [17]. The LifeLink© Log (Table 8-1) is a journal-style log for anecdotal information describing events (both positive and negative) that demonstrate the link between the clinical experience and everyday life. Weekly entries are

TABLE 8-1.
LifeLink© Log with Entry Examples

Date	Entry	Recorder
6/22/94	When asked about his absence on 6/20/94, G.D. explained that a very good friend had lost both his parents on the same day and he had to attend their funeral. G.D. said that the friend had been with him during his difficult days and he had to be supportive when the situation was reversed.	D.L.
		D.L.
6/27/94	G.D. reported to D.L. that he was writing a narrative about his recent experiences for the benefit of other stroke patients.	D.L.
6/29/94	When asked by D.L. to report one incident that made him smile in his daily journal, he commented, "I smile all the time."	D.L.
7/6/94	G.D. reported to D.L. that he had initiated a telephone call for the first time since his stroke. He called his sister.	D.L.

D.L. = a graduate clinician.
Source: B Tucker. Documentation of Quality of Life in Ecological Treatment at the TWU Aphasia Center. [M.A. Professional Paper.] Denton, TX: Texas Woman's University, 1994.

TABLE 8-2.
Critical Questions Used in Structured Interview

What is your typical weekday like?
What is your typical weekend like?
How much are you involved in the decision making in your life?
How do you feel the relationships with other people in your life have changed?
What are your goals for yourself?
What is your satisfaction with life in general?

Source: Adapted from L Hartley. Cognitive-Communicative Abilities following Brain Injury: A Functional Approach. San Diego: Singular Publishing Group, 1995;1–77.

made to record unelicited instances of communication, functional independence, and leisure activity involvement, as well as indicators of psychosocial status. The entries may be directly observed or reported by other clients, volunteers, family members, or transdisciplinary team members. The six critical questions shown in Table 8-2 are asked of the client and significant others at the end of each semester.

TREATMENT GOALS

The speech-language goals for all clients at the Aphasia Center are to establish as much communication ability as possible, establish at least one effective modality for communication, and learn compensatory techniques for residual deficits. Although the Aphasia Center was established for individuals in the chronic stage of recovery, it serves clients at a broad range of time since stroke, varying from 6 weeks to 6 years, and at all levels of severity. Therefore, based on the cumulative assessment results, there are three considerations: (1) level of intervention, (2) intensity of treatment, and (3) specific goals for the client.

Level of Intervention

Level of intervention is a step that places the client on the "recovery-compensation continuum" [19], with linguistic return on one end of the continuum and compensatory techniques on the other end. Most clients are given the opportunity to practice all modalities in the first semester at the Aphasia Center. If the client does not respond to impairment-level treatment, the focus shifts to disability-level treatment. At that level, the goals are to establish at least one effective communication modality and to train compensatory techniques necessary for success in functionally relevant, theme-based communication activities. Clients whose primary problem is at the handicap level receive intervention to lessen the effects of the impairment. They are given opportunities to enhance communicative skills and participate in LifeLink© activities.

Intensity of Intervention

Three levels of treatment are implemented based on the client's severity level on the BDAE (Figure 8-3). Level 1 is comprised of nonverbal communicators with a BDAE severity rating of 1. These clients receive individual speech-language therapy, communication-focused group therapy, psychosocial support for client and family, and LifeLink© activities. Clients with hemiparesis also receive individual assessments and treatment plans from physical and occupational therapy that are implemented at the center. Level 2 is comprised of individuals with limited verbal ability and a BDAE severity rating of 1 or 2. Level 2 clients have been discharged from individual therapy but continue to participate in all other aspects of the program. Level 3 consists of verbal communicators with a BDAE severity rating of 3–5. At level 3, clients participate in client-led discourse groups, are functionally independent, and are encouraged to volunteer at the center and in the community. An alternative treatment program recently developed at the Aphasia Center is the Direct Communication Training Program for family members. In it, an individual program for each client is planned and directly modeled for the family members over an intensive 1-week period. Progress is monitored at regular intervals, and the program is modified as needed.

Specific Goal Setting

Based on the results of the speech-language assessment, the client's current level of function is determined in each modality. Using a general therapeutic hierarchy of task dif-

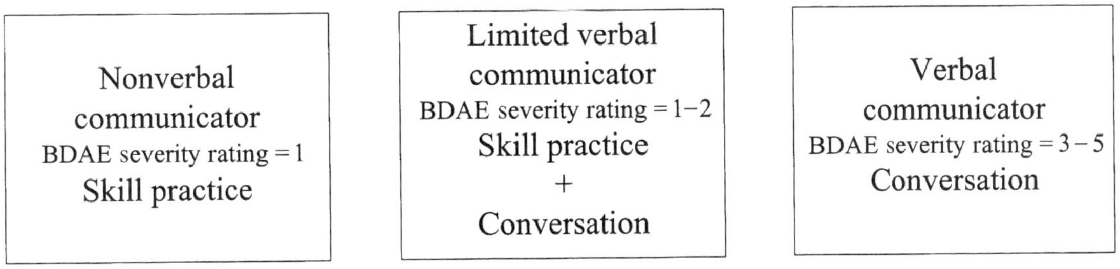

FIGURE 8-3.   **Group levels. (BDAE = Boston Diagnostic Aphasia Examination.)**

ficulty, the current level of performance may be enhanced (i.e., increased efficiency and accuracy) or a higher level task may be targeted.

Transdisciplinary Influence

Because communication treatment occurs within the framework of a transdisciplinary model that generally uses themes as the content and context of treatment, goal setting blends traditional methods with more functionally relevant outcomes based on the current theme. The team establishes a general outcome for each theme, and each discipline does a task analysis to determine prerequisite skills for successful outcome. Based on the client's current abilities, a client-specific goal is established.

CLINICAL TECHNIQUES

Individual Treatment

All clients first participate in individual therapy to (1) re-establish as much language as possible by systematic treatment of all modalities using themes, (2) establish at least one efficient modality for communication, and (3) prepare for communicative success in group and community interactions. Individual therapy goals are addressed using a systematic therapeutic progression that combines traditional and environmentally relevant tasks. Thematically related vocabulary and functional tasks are used as stimuli for treatment regardless of the individualized treatment approach.

Themes

Themes are introduced in individual treatment. The clinician completes an inventory questionnaire with each client to determine level of interest and knowledge about theme. Discussion topics and activities are planned based on this information. Packets of theme-related information are developed and made available to all clinicians for use in individual and group treatment sessions. Each packet contains articles, vocabulary lists, outlines, pictures, and suggested activities. Videotapes related to the themes may also be included. Each clinician is responsible for modifying the content to the severity level of the individual.

Visual Retrieval Language System

We developed an approach we call the Visual Retrieval Language System (VRLS) for use in both individual and group treatment. Initially, this system provides content (theme-related vocabulary) and structure (Fitzgerald key) [20] to facilitate responses (Figure 8-4). At later stages, it provides the structure to extend the length and complex-

ity of utterances. At higher levels of communication ability, discourse outlines are provided. The VRLS is individualized for the client's severity level and is given to the client, allowing for practice in a variety of contexts. Family members are instructed in the use and development of Fitzgerald keys and discourse outlines.

Group Treatment

Group therapy allows clients to implement the skills and strategies that have been a focus of individual speech therapy. Group treatment facilitates generalization or maintenance of communication skills by providing individuals with opportunities to practice communication skills and compensatory strategies in both structured and spontaneous interactions.

Criteria for Forming a Group

Three considerations are important when forming a group: (1) establishing minimal criteria for participation, (2) group size, and (3) homogeneity of group. For individuals to participate successfully in a group, they must be able to follow simple directions and sentence level information; have adequate vision to use the VRLS; be able to read simple, familiar words; and have intact cognitive abilities. The optimal group size is three to five members. When the group has less than three members, interactions often become a series of questions and answers. When the group consists of more than five members, opportunities to communicate are limited. Normal conversation interchanges do not include equal turns by all members, but the purpose of the group experience is to give members as many opportunities as possible to practice communicating.

As described earlier (see Intensity of Intervention), the Aphasia Center has three levels of communication groups, defined by severity on the BDAE (see Figure 8-3). The level of severity determines the amount of structure and direction the speech-language pathologist must provide.

Individuals with a severity rating of 1 on the BDAE participate in skill practice groups. Most individuals in these groups are considered nonverbal communicators. The focus of these groups is skill practice using alternative means of communicating, such as communication notebooks, writing, drawing, and gesturing. The interactions are highly structured, and individuals require maximal support. Individuals with severity rating of 1–2 on the BDAE are placed in groups focusing on skill practice in structured conversations. Interactions are more loosely structured, with the speech-language pathologist providing moderate support. The third level of communication groups is the conversation group. Individuals in these groups are verbal communicators and have a severity rating of 3–5 on the BDAE. This is primarily a client-directed discourse group, with members sharing topic selection with the speech-language pathologist and often assuming complete respon-

Topic

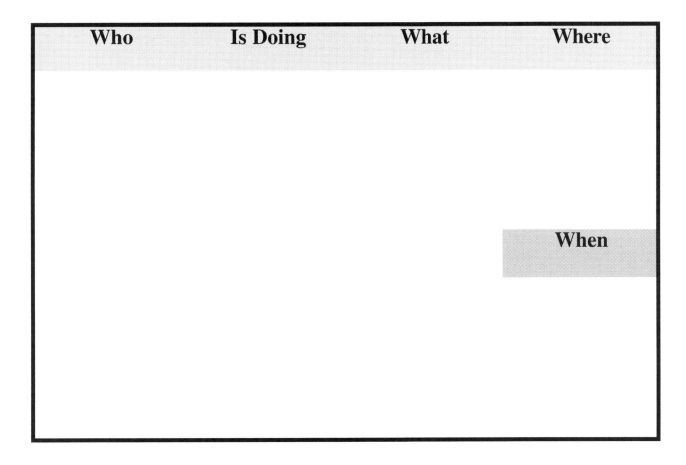

1	2	3	4	5	6	7	8	9	10
11	12	13	14	15	16	17	18	19	20

	0		
10		60	
20		70	
30		80	19_____
40		90	
50		100	

A	B	C	D	E	F
G	H	I	J	K	L
M	N	O	P	Q	R
S	T	U	V	W	
X	Y	Z			

FIGURE 8-4.   **Visual Retrieval Language System: Fitzgerald key.**

sibility for selecting topics for discussion. The speech-language pathologist should act like a group member as much as possible. Participants act as facilitators, and the speech-language pathologist provides minimal support.

Structure of Groups

Group sessions are 75 minutes long and are structured to include the content and time allotted (Table 8-3).

At the beginning of each group session, individual and group goals are reviewed to ensure that all members are aware not only of the group's goals (based on Grice's conversational maxims [21]) but also of one another's individual goals. This review establishes that all members will be active participators, provides them with guidelines to optimize communicative interactions, and establishes their role as facilitators for one another. Facilitation by another individual with aphasia is often much more effective than that by a speech-language pathologist. After the

TABLE 8-3.
Content and Time Allotted in Groups

Length of group therapy session		**1 hour, 15 minutes**
Review goals and strategies		5 minutes
Personal	Ask questions about weekend	10–15 minutes
	Give opportunity to share anything new with other clients	
Current events*	Update or review previous topic	15–30 minutes
	Introduce new topic	
Theme-related activity	Theme: art (e.g., Impressionism)	30–45 minutes
	Discuss artists	
Wrap-up	Discuss overall communication	5–10 minutes
	Use of strategies and facilitation	
	Measure interest in topic or theme using evaluation form	

*Optional.

goals are reviewed, group members engage in social conversation related to personal information (e.g., weekend events, movies, and children) for 10–15 minutes. This conversation is typical of what normally occurs when people get together, and it gives the clinician an opportunity to observe communication skills and collect information to include in the VRLS. The clinician does this by making or adding to previously prepared vocabulary lists, entering vocabulary in Fitzgerald keys, or entering information in narrative discourse outlines. Clients may be able to write some of this information, depending on their severity level. These visuals then provide clients with a way to easily revisit a topic with the same or new listeners. Current events are often discussed in conjunction with or after social conversational time (they are not always included in group). Current events are one of the first themes that clinicians implement at the beginning of each semester. It is an excellent theme to use in introducing the VRLS because it is relevant to most clients and is easily accessible through newspapers, television, and the Internet. Written text, videotapes, and pictures are available through these sources and are easily adapted for use in the VRLS. Clients usually have similar access to current events, so they can provide articles and pictures from personal topics of interest. Current event topics are often ongoing and can be discussed and updated regularly in the group. In addition, they are likely to be topics of discussions in everyday conversations outside the center. Family members who have received instruction in the use of the VRLS facilitate a variety of conversational topics and increase opportunities for communication for the individual with aphasia.

Themes are the central topic of discussion in most groups. Approximately 30–45 minutes are allotted for theme-related activities. If clients have been dismissed from individual therapy, themes are introduced in group therapy. Most themes are implemented for a minimum of 2 weeks, but they can be extended or expanded as need or interest dictates. Theme-related group activities include discussions, debates, role-play, problem-solving activities, and planning activities for the LifeLink© program. The VRLS is used to facilitate communication and to optimize the interaction. Higher-level communication groups frequently select their own topics or themes. Some groups have elected to do book

or movie reviews, discuss possible or favorite vacation places, or focus on a current event of interest. During the last 10–15 minutes of group therapy, clients evaluate their performance by completing an evaluation form about interest in topic, frequency of opportunities to communicate, their success in communicating, and how the clinician communicated with them (e.g., rate of speech, complexity of language). This gives the clinician and the group members a means to discuss communication and solve any problems. This ending period is usually a very positive experience, allowing members to brag about one another's skills.

DISCHARGE CRITERIA

The Aphasia Center is a community of people with shared experiences, so it is our philosophy that clients be allowed to continue in LifeLink© activities for as long as they wish to do so. However, when it is determined by the professional staff that an individual has recovered maximum benefit from individual speech therapy, treatment is terminated but the client may remain in group or LifeLink© activities. Clients who become nonparticipatory or too fragile medically may be discharged. As clients progress and begin to expand their community life, self-discharge is likely. Several clients have completed their time as clients and returned as volunteers.

Volunteers

The Aphasia Center has a small volunteer component that complements our program. Volunteers include previous clients, clients currently at the center, family members, and individuals from the community. Client volunteers serve primarily as communication partners to other clients and assist them in communication during center and community activities. Family members and community volunteers offer their talents and time by teaching specialty classes (e.g., art, woodwork, and golf) or by assisting in planning and implementing LifeLink© activities. We encourage family members to limit their volunteer time, using the time that clients are at the center as respite time for themselves.

REIMBURSEMENT ISSUES

The Aphasia Center currently charges $150 for the initial intake assessment and a minimal semester fee of $300. Clients who receive individual physical therapy are charged an additional fee of $150. Most fees are paid for privately because medical insurance benefits have been depleted for hospitalization or rehabilitation. We have limited scholarship funding for clients who need financial assistance.

REFERENCES

1. Friedland JF, McColl M. Social support intervention after stroke: results of a randomized trial. Arch Phys Med Rehabil 1992;73:573–581.
2. Simmons NN. A trip down easy street. Clin Aphasiol 1992;19:19–30.
3. Lyon J. Communicative use and participation in life for aphasic adults in natural settings: the scope of the problem. Am J Speech Lang Pathol 1992;1[3]:7–14.
4. Hartley L. Cognitive-Communicative Abilities following Brain Injury: A Functional Approach. San Diego: Singular Publishing Group, 1995;1–77.
5. Lubinski R. Environmental Language Intervention. In R Chapey (ed), Language Intervention Strategies in Adults. Baltimore: Williams & Wilkins, 1981;23–45.
6. Merzenich MM, Kass JH, Wall J, et al. Topographic reorganization of somatosensory cortical areas 3B and 1 in adult monkeys following restricted differentiation. Neuroscience 1983;8:33–55.
7. Goodglass H, Kaplan E. The Boston Diagnostic Aphasia Examination. In The Assessment of Aphasia and Related Disorders. Philadelphia: Lea & Febiger, 1983;29–50.
8. Helms-Estabrook N, Ramsberger G, Morgan A, Nicholas M. The Boston Assessment of Severe Aphasia. Chicago: Riverside, 1992.
9. Darley FL, Aronson AE, Brown JR. Motor Speech Disorders. Philadelphia: Saunders, 1975;86–98.
10. Helms-Estabrook N. Test of Oral and Limb Apraxia. Chicago: Riverside, 1992.
11. Frattali CM, Thompson CK, Holland AI, et al. Functional Assessment of Communication Skills for Adults (ASHA FACS). Rockville, MD: ASHA, 1995.
12. Overs RP. Avocational Activities Inventory. Presented at Curative Workshop of Milwaukee, Milwaukee, WI, 1971.
13. Niklas M, Dickerson S. Assessment of Quality of Life Changes in Ecological Treatment at the TWU Aphasia Center. A Pilot Study. [M.A. Professional Paper.] Denton, TX: Texas Woman's University, 1995.
14. Stern RA, Hooper C. Stern and Hooper Visual Analogue Mood Scales. [Unpublished manuscript.] Chapel Hill, NC: University of North Carolina Department of Psychiatry, 1991.
15. McNair DM, Lorr M, Dropleman LF. Profile of Mood States (rev ed). San Diego: Educational and Industrial Testing Service, 1981.
16. Clarke SF. Assessment of Psychosocial Well Being and Depression in Aphasic Families. [M.A. Professional Paper.] Denton, TX: Texas Woman's University, 1993.
17. Ryff CD. Happiness is everything, or is it? Explorations on the meaning of psychological well being. J Pers Soc Psychol 1989;57:1069–1081.
18. Tucker B. Documentation of Quality of Life in Ecological Treatment at the TWU Aphasia Center. [M.A. Professional Paper.] Denton TX: Texas Woman's University, 1994.
19. Elman R. Aphasia Treatment Planning in an Outpatient Medical Rehabilitation Center: Where Do We Go from Here? In C Coehlo (ed), Neurophysiology and Neurogenic Speech and Language Disorders Special Interest Division 2 Newsletter. Rockville, MD: American Speech-Language Hearing Association, 1994;9–13.
20. Fitzgerald G. Straight Language for the Deaf: A System of Instructions for Deaf Children (2nd ed). Austin, TX: Eck Co, 1937.
21. Grice H. Logic and Conversation. In P Cole (ed), Syntax and Semantics. Speech Acts, vol. 3. New York: Academic Press, 1975.
22. Fugl-Meyer A, Jaasko L, Leyman I, et al. The post-stroke hemiplegic patient: a method of evaluation of physical performance. Scand J Rehabil Med 1975;7:13–31.
23. Mathias S, Nayak USL, Isaacs B. Balance in elderly patients: the "get-up-and-go" test. Arch Phys Med Rehabil 1986;67:387.
24. Mahoney FI, Barthel DW. Functional evaluation: the Barthel Index. Maryland State Med J 1965;14:61–65.
25. Law M, Baptiste S, Carswell A, et al. Canadian Occupational Performance Measure. Ottawa: CAOT Publications, 1994.
26. Yesage JA, Brink TL, Rose TL, et al. Development and validation of a geriatric depression screening scale: a preliminary report. J Psychiatr Res 1983;17:37–49.

CHAPTER NINE

Aphasia Groups: The Arizona Experience

Audrey L. Holland and
Pelagie M. Beeson

PHILOSOPHY OF THE PROGRAM

One of the greatest losses experienced by people with aphasia is the reduced opportunity for everyday conversation. Because conversation is so pervasive and so interactional, its disturbance can be devastating. We rely on spoken language to make requests, to make our wants and needs known, and to provide information. We also use language to connect with people, to interact, and to enjoy each other. For example, when you enter a cab and tell the driver your destination, and he gets you there, you have successfully negotiated an interpersonal transaction. If on the way to your destination, you chat with the driver about politics, traffic, or your hometown, you have enjoyed the interactional aspects of communication. People with aphasia experience failure to communicate and disrupted social interaction. Our aphasia groups were designed to provide opportunities to re-establish interaction at verbal and non-verbal levels in a setting that promotes success.

Our goals at the University of Arizona Aphasia Clinic are threefold: (1) to facilitate successful communication despite residual language impairment, (2) to encourage communication using all modalities, and (3) to teach and elaborate specific communication strategies. We believe that many benefits derive from aphasia groups conceptualized in this manner; they range from decreasing social isolation to establishing and maintaining supportive friendships to providing an opportunity to laugh along with people who understand your problems.

In this chapter, we describe the formal characteristics of our aphasia groups and provide specific examples of successful activities undertaken in our groups. The role of a group facilitator, and the training necessary to become one, are also covered. We discuss our services for family members, our experiences in developing aphasia groups, and some ideas about how others might profitably proceed in this undertaking.

CHARACTERISTICS OF THE PROGRAM

Although we have often been tempted to diversify, we have concentrated our efforts on individuals with a history of left hemisphere stroke. We have no doubt that group experience has a role in the rehabilitation of individuals with right hemisphere stroke, but we believe that the requisite group experience for them would differ greatly from what appears to help people with aphasia. It is clear that group experiences for individuals with head injury are beneficial, and there is a richer history of such groups than exists for aphasic individuals [1]. We chose to focus on aphasia because we lack the resources (e.g., personnel, space, time) to undertake group treatment for other acquired neurogenic disorders.

We provide service to roughly 40 individuals with aphasia and their caregivers every Friday. The ages of group members have ranged from 28 to 89. Members also vary widely in length of time post-onset, ranging from 1 month to 14 years. Although conversation groups are the central focus, some

group members receive individual therapy as well. Currently, eight groups are scheduled for 1-hour sessions during the course of the day. We have learned that groups function best when they are small; most groups have five to seven participants to maximize the time spent talking by each group member. One advantage of a relatively large program such as ours is that we have been able to build groups with people who have similar levels of communication ability. This makes it easier to select appropriate activities. It is also easier to balance talking time when severity is relatively homogeneous. However, we are not particularly motivated to determine group membership by type of aphasia; in fact, it is relatively commonplace for us to include both fluent and nonfluent talkers in the same group. Mixing people with different forms of aphasia appears to work well. Nonfluent members appear to tolerate the excessive output of fluent members, and the telegraphic output of some agrammatic speakers is relatively easy for other group members to understand. Other factors that influence group placement are level of education, previous vocation, and range and type of interests. For example, in one of our groups all members but two had lived abroad for an extensive period and were fluent in at least one language besides English.

All conversation groups are facilitated by clinical and research faculty and graduate students. Therefore, the clinic naturally runs for fall, spring, and summer terms that coincide with the academic schedule. Sessions are scheduled for an hour, but sometimes groups run longer, depending on needs and the available space. On occasion, groups extend their time together by going out to lunch after a session, and a few "group groupies" actively participate in more than one group. Sessions are staggered throughout the day, making it unlikely that the 60-odd members, caretakers, and clinicians are all in the clinic at the same time, although we do have occasional parties and sessions for the entire membership. Very few group members come at the appointed hour and then leave promptly. Quirks of the handicapped transportation system of Tucson aside, aphasic members and their caretakers often come early, perhaps to munch on the goodies (low-fat, diabetic) that are always available, but more typically to hang out, catch up, and develop relationships.

For some members, the group aids transition from individual treatment at one of the local hospitals to eventual dismissal from therapy. More commonly, members have a long-term affiliation. Far from discouraging such long-term involvement, groups are often essential for maintaining aphasic people's use of compensatory communication strategies and for meeting their psychosocial needs. The group itself seems to function as what Kagan calls a "communication ramp," supporting and providing access to social interaction that seems lacking in the rest of the aphasic person's world [2].

WHAT HAPPENS IN APHASIA GROUPS?

The groups have many facets and serve many purposes. Here are some of them:

1. We provide both direct and indirect language treatment.
2. We encourage and model the use of a variety of communication strategies.
3. We offer psychosocial support in both planned and spontaneous ways for members and their families.
4. We provide continual education to patients and families and to our student-clinicians as well.

Kearns [3] provided a comprehensive review of approaches to group treatment, but it is difficult to capture the dynamics of a group activity on paper. In what follows, we give detailed descriptions of activities we have found useful. Before we begin, it is important to acknowledge that overall severity of aphasia plays a role in dictating our group activities. For moderate and high-level groups, activities such as personal updates and conversations on hot topics, problem solving, life planning, decision making, and coping with aphasia are often easier than they are for moderately severe and severe groups. More impaired groups often require direction from the facilitator to initiate and maintain conversation.

Clinical Techniques to Evoke Group Conversation

Conversation mostly just happens. Being summoned to a conversation is essentially an oxymoron, conjuring up memories of being told to "Go talk to your Aunt Emma now" or "Tell Mr. Jones all about your fishing trip." For members with milder disabilities, many topics of conversation simply come up naturally. Planning is minimal, and talk flows in many directions. Personal highlights of the past week, interesting news events, celebrity gossip, assignments given by one group member to another—essentially what individuals wish to share with each other—always take precedence over carefully developed plans (especially when the plans are developed by clinicians). We have found this laissez-faire approach to be difficult, almost threatening, for neophyte group facilitators, but it is perfectly within the purview of a successful aphasia group session.

Our goal is for group members to succeed in conversation independent of the modality they are required to use. By selecting topics that are likely to emerge in everyday conversation, group sessions serve as practice for conversations outside the clinic. Many topics recur in conversation groups. These include current events (particularly the more controversial), what's new in someone's life, previous occupations and places lived before, family, travel, sports, and hobbies. No clinician should approach an aphasia group without having looked at the latest *People* magazine. We have even found an excuse for our grocery-line habit of reading the *National Enquirer* ("Just getting ready for aphasia group!"). Student clinicians probably need to read the newspaper or at least watch a morning news show to keep up with our group members' knowledge of current events.

Independent of the severity of aphasia, several important principles are paramount for group success. First, conversation requires sharing. Both aphasic and non-aphasic facilitators must participate in receiving and providing information, feelings, reactions, and opinions. For example, imagine the relative effectiveness of a session designed to talk about one's most embarrassing moment in which the facilitator begins by saying, "We're going to talk about our most embarrassing moments today. Bob, do you want to begin?" and "I had the most embarrassing experience of my life today. Let me tell you about it." At best, the first approach will draw minimal responses. At worst, the second will draw a good laugh, but it is also very likely to turn into a "Can you top this?" session.

Ideally, conversational discussions are also initiated by group members. A particularly poignant exchange occurred in one of our groups when Mr. M tearfully told us that a neighbor had accused him of breaking into his house. The misunderstanding arose because Mr. M was trying to tell the neighbor that he had seen their dog running loose. The neighbor did not understand Mr. M's gestures or his perseverative utterance "1, 2, 3," and thus assumed the worst. Sharing this story required Mr. M to use all possible communication modes: drawing, gesturing, writing, and emotion-laden perseverative utterances. His successful conveyance drew great empathy from group members and led to the discussion of other aphasia-related dramas.

Group facilitators also strive for levity, laughter, and a heavy dose of good humor. As rapport develops, the opportunity for verbal and nonverbal joking grows. Finding ways to enjoy life again is a major factor in reducing the handicap of aphasia, and, as Kagan suggested [2,4], so is the opportunity to forget for a while that one has this frustrating disorder. Laughter is not reserved for our most recovered groups. One of our most cherished videotapes shows one globally aphasic person catching another member of his group as he makes a mistake in counting spaces in a board game or, possibly, cheating. The first person quickly and physically corrected the "mistake," through exaggeration, and comically signaled his disapproval. Then, both men reached out to each other and shared a good deep laugh.

This vignette foreshadows what is probably the most important benefit of group therapy. Support, in myriad forms, is the essential ingredient of aphasia groups. Some support is clinician-driven and consists of skillful use of many helpful communication devices. Examples include using written choices to facilitate successful communication [5]; serving as a "communication broker," that is, seeking and confirming each piece of information to make sure it is understandable to other group members; prompting members in the use of potentially successful communication strategies to supplant or augment their speaking attempts; and providing a model of communication accompanied by gesture, drawing, and writing. Although we encourage direct communication among group members, we recognize that we are asking aphasic speakers to decode the aphasic communication of other group members. That is sometimes unrealistic, and the facilitator must always be prepared to take an active role in a group's communication exchange. In many instances, group members directly encourage communication attempts and even motivate one another to try new communication strategies.

By far, the most critical aspect of support in aphasia groups is the psychosocial support provided by others who are walking in "aphasia moccasins." We do not specifically structure sessions to be support groups. Nonetheless, group members take the opportunity to vent and to share frustrations and concerns with one another. Because our groups include individuals at different stages of adjustment to the impact of stroke and aphasia, they often serve as role models for the process of recovery. The spirit of camaraderie that permits aphasia groups to be lively and light, of course, also makes it possible for aphasic individuals to share their collective losses, to mourn what is gone, and to provide true empathy.

Group Activities

Other activities of our groups encompass various aspects of communication. The sample provided here is far from exhaustive, and we do not intend to stifle readers' imagination and creativity by highlighting only a few topics.

1. Role playing and simulations. Aphasia group members sometimes have concerns about the communication demands of an upcoming event. In such cases, role playing is useful. Group members can practice getting rid of unwanted telephone solicitors, shopping, taking the dog to the veterinarian, and so forth. In some cases, actual "scripts" are developed and practiced by group members to help them communicate important life stories. In his discussion of problem-focused activities for group treatment, Marshall [6] provides a number of other examples (see also Chapter 7).

2. Memory books. Another potentially successful activity, particularly for more severely impaired individuals, is the construction of memory books, as described by Bourgeois [7]. Although she intended such books to be used with memory-impaired individuals, they clearly have utility in some aphasia groups. Memory books, which chronicle individual life events through photographs and captions, provide stimulating information to conversational partners both in and out of the clinic. It is important for aphasic people to be able to present themselves not simply as aphasic people but as they have been through most of their lives. Self-respect might demand that they share their histories, accomplishments, and dreams. Memory books can be helpful in communicating who one is, beneath the aphasia. We have discovered many fascinating aspects to the lives of many patients by having shared their newspaper clippings, awards, and photograph albums.

3. Promoting Aphasic Communicative Effectiveness (PACE). Many of our activities are based on the principles of PACE. Davis and Wilcox [8] introduced PACE as an individual treatment procedure to encourage communication using all modalities in an authentic

manner. In PACE activities, (a) new information is exchanged, (b) any mode of communication is acceptable, (c) both partners are senders and receivers of information, and (d) feedback is that of the real world—being understood or not. Springer [9] provided guidelines for using PACE in groups. In a group of severely aphasic members, for example, the goal might be for one member of the group to communicate to others (e.g., by drawing, gesture) the name of a famous person whose picture he is looking at but withholding from others. Group members attempt to guess, possibly also with gestures or drawings. Feedback is the success (or failure) of communicating. PACE sessions may be highly competitive and provide excellent confirmation of the utility or worthlessness of particular strategies, or the power of using multiple strategies simultaneously. Context can be structured to enhance relevance to everyday communication, and group PACE activities can be adapted across a wide range of severity levels.

4. Stating opinions and solving problems. Group discussion that centers on stating opinions and solving problems is a natural parallel to nonaphasic conversation. Problems can range from the hypothetical ("My neighbor's unmarried daughter just found out she is pregnant. What should she do?") to the potentially real and certainly interesting ("What would you do if you won the Arizona Lottery, worth $5 million?") to the very real and important ("How can we share the message about the importance of aphasia groups?"). We have ample evidence that aphasia rarely diminishes one's power to hold opinions and, with enough communication support, to voice them. Therefore, activities centered on expressing opinions and consequent actions are productive and healthy.

5. Games. We occasionally use card or board games, particularly in our more severely impaired groups, but with the strong caution that communication goals must be kept in mind. That is, just playing a quiet game may be enjoyable, but it does not satisfy communication goals. Some games, such as Pictionary or Scrabble, require little adaptation for successful group application. Others, such as Taboo, are easily adaptable and can be used to practice alternative communicative strategies, such as gesture or drawing.

GROUP FACILITATOR RESPONSIBILITIES

We have been careful to use *facilitator* to describe the non-aphasic person who is responsible for implementing group process. *Leader* seems inappropriate and too laden with authority. Among the responsibilities of the facilitator are these:

1. Facilitating conversations or activities. This requires advance planning, even if the ensuing session "just

happens," as described earlier. Facilitators must ensure that paper, markers, and maps are always available. If conversation or interaction is not forthcoming, the facilitator must take up the slack. To maximize comprehension, the facilitator may confirm or clarify information in a natural way so that meaning becomes clear to other group members.

2. Maximizing communication effectiveness. The role of information broker is important here. The facilitator must establish appropriate expectations for individual group members, set the example of accepting communication through all modalities, and structure tasks appropriate to members' abilities.

3. Promoting increased group independence. The facilitator encourages member-initiated discussion and prompts group members to share. One must always keep a watchful eye out for members who may wish to participate but need encouragement, even an invitation, to do so. Serving as a role model for group members in facilitating interchange is an important responsibility. Perhaps the most difficult aspect of promoting independence is for the facilitator to learn to reduce involvement, to keep quiet, as group members increase their participation.

4. Teaching. Facilitators must identify effective and ineffective strategies for each group member and, in some cases, directly teach or model strategies that work. For example, one of our group members effectively used gestures to give meaning to his fluent jargon, but he rarely attempted to write. We saw that he had the potential to write some single words (or the first few letters of some words), so he was coached in the group setting to supplement his gestures with attempts at writing a word or a letter. This combined strategy led to improved communication for proper names in particular, such as writing N__ J___ to communicate his home state of New Jersey. Conversely, another group member frequently attempted to write single words that rarely, if ever, provided useful information, because they were off-target and perseverative. She was guided to use gestures and simple drawings to supplement her empty verbal output, resulting in greater communicative success. The group environment is ideal for discerning and establishing optimal use of communication strategies.

5. Encouraging and nurturing support within the group. There are many common issues of concern to most aphasia groups. These include driving, medication, seizures, disability insurance, work status and opportunities, and changed family roles, to cite a few. Aphasia groups are appropriate arenas for their discussion, and the leader must create a climate for sharing problems as well as solutions.

6. Setting the tone. Facilitators have the primary role in setting the tone of groups. It is important to strive for a caring and respectful environment, where friendships can transcend political or religious differences. Moreover, the attitude should be upbeat and centered on moving forward in life.

FAMILY GROUPS

We believe that the needs of family members are likely to be as great as the needs of aphasic individuals themselves. Therefore, we also conduct separate groups for family members. They are variously run by faculty members, psychologists, graduate clinical psychology interns, and social workers. Family groups deal with a number of issues involving both education and support. Surprisingly, the topics of stroke and related medical issues never seem to grow old, and we frequently revisit them from different vantage points. Two or three times a year, our family groups profit from an opportunity to meet with a neurologist to re-establish their basic understanding of stroke and stroke recovery. Topics such as seizures and physical rehabilitation frequently appear on the educational agenda of family groups. We also invite travel agents to talk about handicapped traveling tips, dietitians to talk about how to count fat grams, and audiologists to talk about hearing impairments.

The support function of family groups is as important as it is in aphasia groups themselves. Family groups provide opportunities for grieving and for expressing guilt, feelings of depression, and concerns about being overprotective or not protective enough. As new members join family groups, more experienced ones provide mentoring, modeling, and the sage advice that comes from experience. We have had sessions on topics as disparate as giving ridiculously simple recipes to the husband of a newly aphasic woman who said he could only heat TV dinners, and talking through the fears and concerns that are a major part of living with individuals who have aphasia.

As with aphasic individuals themselves, lifestyle changes occur for family members, particularly partners. Social isolation is common, and reduced opportunities for social interaction are almost inevitable. Ironically, the spouse's plight is often invisible, even to children who are counting on Mom to be there for Dad but are not aware that aphasia also has a very direct impact on Mom. Thus, there are many important issues for family groups, but there are rewards as well. For example, family members often forge lasting friendships and strong social bonds.

In our clinic, family group participation is voluntary. A few spouses never come; others never fail to show up. Some enterprising spouses view aphasia group time as respite; one spouse consistently chooses a manicure over our ministrations. On one occasion, we observed two wives, frequent attendees at the spouse group, leaving the building immediately after having delivered their husbands to group. Thinking they had failed to note that spouse group was about to start, we commented. Giggling and blushing like schoolgirls playing hooky, they confessed that they had decided to steal away for a few hours of shopping and had certainly not intended to get caught. We wished them well and waved them on.

TRAINING OF GROUP FACILITATORS

The traditional training of most speech-language pathologists is inadequate preparation for facilitating aphasia groups. Skills in group and interpersonal communication are desirable, as is knowledge of aphasia and its management. Our approach to training students is to work with them side by side in the group setting while we provide a model for them. Assigned readings include an article about talking to individuals with aphasia by Holland and Halper [10]. Students are required to watch Aphasia Group Telerounds [11], as well as the Pat Arato Aphasia Centre's recent videotape on supported communication [4]. We encourage students to be videotaped in conversational interaction with aphasic individuals and then provide play-by-play critiques as we watch them together. When students are reticent to participate so directly, training is provided via videotapes of others being trained, again with accompanying critique.

We never assign a beginning student to run an aphasia group alone. A student might function as an assistant for several weeks, learning the skills by observation. Feedback is given after every session, and plans for the next session are reviewed. As the term goes on, student clinicians assume an increasingly larger facilitative role. Learning group dynamics as well as how to talk to and understand individuals with aphasia are essentially new skills for our students. It takes guidance, patience, and talent for a student to become comfortable with this role. We believe that training is essentially similar for students, volunteers, speech-language pathology aides, physicians, and other health care personnel who wish to be maximally effective in communicating with aphasic adults.

STARTING AN APHASIA GROUP PROGRAM

The topic of how to start an aphasia group program probably demands its own chapter or a detailed manual. Nonetheless, we can make some basic points. Once one decides to start a group, some important steps inevitably must be taken. Our best advice is to start small and accommodate growth as it occurs. It is necessary to be flexible at the outset and to anticipate change. When we started our groups, we identified a list of potential group members by informing fellow professionals at acute care and rehabilitation centers in the Tucson area about our decision to start groups. We also informed agencies and associations, such as the local chapters of the American Heart Association, the Easter Seal Society, and the National Aphasia Association. Most of our referrals come from community-based speech-language pathologists, although one member was referred by her hairdresser! We have cast a wide net, and like the hero of the movie *Field of Dreams*, we believe that "If you build it, they will come."

Our clinic operates in the midst of a busy multipurpose speech and language clinic. Adequate parking and handicapped accessibility are necessities. We work in small rooms, with group meetings taking place at round tables, whenever possible. Minimum equipment includes notepads, markers, maps, tissues, and some source of hot water for beverages. (We yearn for superb and simple augmentative devices, cupboards full of wonderful and appropriate games, menus from every restaurant in town, and videotaping and computer facilities in every treatment room.)

Entry and Discharge Criteria

Having aphasia constitutes our admission criteria. We conduct an interview and initial assessment, but we have rarely turned away potential group members because their aphasia is too severe or too mild. We maintain a waiting list but usually manage to squeeze in patients in a relatively short time. We have no dismissal criteria. The four most likely ways to terminate one's relationship with our program are to die, to move, to determine that one's needs have been met, or to decide that the group's cost-benefit ratio has been exceeded. Less common, but excellent, reasons that members leave our group include returning to work or starting their own aphasia group. We have only once asked a member to leave: He was one of our oldest members, his aphasia was increasingly overshadowed by dementia, and his participation in group became disruptive. Although we dismissed him from group, his spouse continued her involvement in the family group. Other group members have declined cognitively or physically, thereby precluding the feasibility of group participation, but those members and their families recognized their changing status, making it unnecessary to initiate dismissal.

Reimbursement Issues

Financial considerations are very real. Aphasia groups are not a way for speech-language pathologists to become rich. We are fortunate to be housed in a university clinic, which makes financial considerations possibly less urgent than for clinicians in other settings. Few members have insurance benefits that cover our services, largely because most of them are so long post-stroke. Nonetheless, group treatment is reimbursable in many states.

As our clinic has developed, our point of view about payment for group services has evolved. Many people (including aphasic patients and their families) are willing to pay for services simply because those services make them feel good. Some examples include aerobics classes, massages, or having shirts laundered professionally. In these cases, third-party reimbursement is never an issue. Group treatment for aphasia might well be considered one of these services, and they are marketed to potential members as having such benefits. This makes self-pay more palatable, particularly given that group treatment

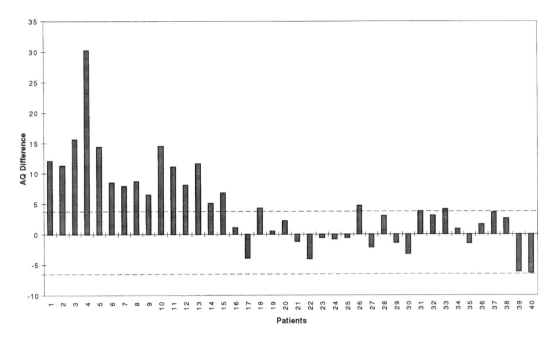

FIGURE 9-1.

Change in Western Aphasia Battery aphasia quotients (AQ) for 40 individuals before and after aphasia group participation. Note that 15 individuals showed improved AQ scores of 5 or greater, 23 remained relatively stable, and 2 individuals showed a decline of more than 5 AQ points.

fees can be considerably lower than individual treatment fees. The astute clinician should recognize that the time spent on reimbursement paperwork is obviated, thereby freeing up more hours for more groups. In such a climate, it is perfectly reasonable to include an occasional indigent client or invoke a sliding fee scale.

LONG-TERM OUTCOMES

Our groups were designed to maximize communication abilities, and we expected group members to improve their communication skills in very functional ways. We hoped they would learn to be more flexible in choosing a communication modality, be more persistent and successful in their attempts to convey meaning, feel more comfortable working around their persistent language impairment, and strengthen a new sense of self [12]. All these things have happened: We can see it, family members attest to it, and a few of our patients have even written about it [13–15].

The rich anecdotal evidence that many patients were improving was complemented by yearly formal assessments of language abilities. Our data showed that many group members continued to make significant gains long after the first few months post-stroke, which has been identified as the period of greatest recovery [16]. Our data are restricted in that we did not have a prospective study in place and there was no matched control group who did not participate in group treatment. Additionally, our group members varied depending on whether they

also received individual therapy. Despite these caveats, our longitudinal data have helped us describe the long-term outcomes of individual group members, helped to shape our expectations for other patients, and guided our family counseling.

We collected longitudinal data from 40 members of our aphasia groups who joined at various times post-onset, ranging from 3 months to 14 years (mean = 2.8 years, standard deviation [SD] = 3.3 years). There were 29 men and 11 women, with an average age at the time of stroke of 59.7 years (SD = 15.6 years). All participated in an aphasia group for at least 1 calendar year and were tested at yearly intervals with the Western Aphasia Battery (WAB) [17]. We examined the changes in each group member's WAB aphasia quotient (AQ) over time. In Figure 9-1, we show the difference in AQ scores from the time each member joined the group to their most recent WAB, which was an average interval of 2.4 years.

Three performance patterns were observed: (1) those who made significant language improvement (defined as an increase of at least 5 AQ points [18]); (2) those who made no significant change in language performance (an AQ ±5 points of initial testing); and (3) those who showed a significant decline in language performance (a drop in AQ of more than 5 points). Of 40 group members, 15 (37.5%) showed significant language improvement as measured by the WAB, 23 (57.5%) showed no significant change in AQ, and two (5%) showed a significant decline in AQ. We found these data encouraging in that more than one-third of our group members showed continued measurable language improvement during a period when they would be considered to have chronic aphasia.

An examination of the data suggested that the people whose language significantly improved tended to be younger and have more recent post-onset times than those who did not change, but these differences were not statistically significant. A regression equation was calculated to determine if age at onset of stroke, time post-onset, or the time elapsed between the WAB examinations were significant predictors of language improvement. The regression equation was significant (f(37) = 5.046, *P* = .012), with age at time of stroke and time post-onset being the significant predictor variables. We interpret these results to mean that younger patients who had their strokes more recently had a slightly better recovery outlook than older patients who were longer post-onset. The regression equation accounted for only 21% of the variance, however, suggesting that many other factors also influence language improvement.

The majority of our patients did not show significant improvement on the WAB. In other words, most of our patients showed relatively fixed language impairments. Our anecdotal evidence suggested that many of those group members became better communicators as they used more effective communication strategies; however, we await confirmation from our longitudinal testing on functional measures of communication [19].

We were not surprised by the performance of the two individuals whose AQs significantly declined during their last year of group affiliation. Both were in their seventies and had other age-related medical problems while their language was declining. Although neither experienced a new clinically documented stroke, one of these individuals died from a cardiovascular event several months after his last WAB, and the other became homebound within the year due to health decline. We have been working with post-stroke patients long enough to recognize this pattern of decline in older, relatively unhealthy individuals with aphasia. The pattern consists of a long period of language improvement or steady-state performance followed by decline that appears to reflect the aging of a lesioned brain.

CONCLUSION

We are enthusiastic about group treatment for aphasic individuals. We believe that group experiences offer challenge and hope to aphasic people that are not otherwise available. Earlier in this chapter, we discussed the need to be flexible while developing groups. We also believe that continued flexibility is equally important. Our ideas are not cast in concrete; they merely indicate where our experiences have led us at this particular moment. We expect our concepts of group management to change and become more sophisticated as more clinicians undertake group treatment and thereby increase knowledge of this particularly exciting development in clinical aphasiology.

Acknowledgments

The information provided in this chapter reflects what our aphasia group members have taught us. We thank them for these lessons and for their patience as we try to get it right.

This work was supported, in part, by National Multipurpose Research and Training Center Grant DC-01409 from the National Institute on Deafness and Other Communication Disorders.

REFERENCES

1. Ylvisaker M, Holland A. Coaching, Self-Coaching, and Recovery from Head Injury. In D Johns (ed), Clinical Management of Neurogenic Communication Disorders (rev ed). Boston: Little, Brown, 1985.
2. Kagan A. Revealing the competence of aphasic adults through conversation: a challenge to health professionals. Top Stroke Rehabil 1995;2:15–27.
3. Kearns KP. Group Therapy for Aphasia: Theoretical and Practical Considerations. In R Chapey (ed), Language Intervention Strategies in Adult Aphasia (3rd ed). Baltimore: Williams & Wilkins, 1994;304–321.
4. Kagan A, Shumway E. Supported Conversation for Aphasic Adults. North York, Ontario: Aphasia Centre of North York, 1996.
5. Garrett KL. Written choice conversation: a treatment technique for severe aphasia. Presented at the Annual Convention of the American Speech-Language-Hearing Association, Anaheim, CA, November 1993.
6. Marshall RC. Problem-focused group therapy for mildly aphasic clients. Am J Speech Lang Pathol 1993;2:31–37.
7. Bourgeois MS. Conversing with Memory-Impaired Individuals Using Memory Aids: A Memory Aid Workbook. Gaylord, MI: Northern Speech Services, 1992.
8. Davis GA, Wilcox MJ. Incorporating Parameters of Natural Conversation in Aphasia Treatment. In R Chapey (ed), Language Intervention Strategies in Adult Aphasia. Baltimore: Williams & Wilkins, 1981.
9. Springer L. Facilitating group rehabilitation. Aphasiology 1991; 6:563–565.
10. Holland AL, Halper AS. Talking to individuals with aphasia: a challenge for the rehabilitation team. Top Stroke Rehabil 1996;2:27–37.
11. Beeson PM, Holland AL. Telerounds No. 19: Aphasia Groups: An Approach to Long-Term Rehabilitation. Tucson, AZ: National Center for Neurogenic Communication Disorders, September 1994.
12. Holland AL, Beeson PM. Finding a new sense of self: what the clinician can do to help. A reply to Brumfitt's "Losing one's sense of self after stroke." Aphasiology 1993;7:569–591.
13. Ross R. Aphasia groups. Advance for Speech-Language Pathologists & Audiologists 1996;6(19):18–19.
14. Moore DE. A second start. Top Stroke Rehabil 1994;1:100–103.
15. Vail SM. Survivor recounts "painful, bewildering" experience with stroke. Advance for Speech-Language Pathologists & Audiologists 1997;7(28):18–19.
16. Kertesz A. Recovery from Aphasia. In TE Feinberg, MJ Farah (eds), Behavioral Neurology and Neuropsychology. New York: McGraw-Hill, 1997;167–182.
17. Kertesz A. Western Aphasia Battery. New York: Grune & Stratton, 1982.
18. Shewan CM, Kertesz A. Reliability and validity characteristics of the Western Aphasia Battery (WAB). J Speech Hear Disord 1980;45:308–324.
19. Frattali CM, Thompson CK, Holland AL, et al. American Speech-Language-Hearing Association Functional Assessment of Communication Skills for Adults. Rockville, MD: American Speech-Language-Hearing Association, 1995.

CHAPTER TEN

Group Communication Therapy for People with Long-Term Aphasia: Scaffolded Thematic Discourse Activities

Kathryn L. Garrett
and Gayle J. Ellis

This chapter presents a model of group language intervention for people with long-term aphasia developed in 1994 at the University of Nebraska–Lincoln Speech Language and Hearing Clinic [1]. The primary purpose of the intervention program was to provide continuing opportunities for people with long-term aphasia to improve their communication skills in integrative contexts. The model also was developed as a teaching vehicle for graduate students in speech-language pathology who were delivering group therapy services in the Speech and Hearing Clinic.

In the Nebraska model, principles of discourse, thematicity (or the centralization of information related to a particular concept or event), contextual support, and functional use are integrated throughout group communication activities. Four instructional phases (conversation, context building, language mediation, and final discourse activity) provide a continuum of deep language intervention to prepare each individual to participate maximally in relevant conversational and thematic discourse activities. Specific communication skills (e.g., attention and comprehension, semantic specificity, organization of discourse, social-pragmatic skills, use of compensatory communication strategies, and reading or writing) are targeted for all participants. Clinicians provide ongoing scaffolding and instructional support using methods based on principles of information organization, communication opportunities, and provision of natural and meaningful feedback discussed by Norris and Hoffman [2]. Throughout the activities, and after completing the final discourse activities, people engage in self-evaluation of their communication performance.

RATIONALE

Group Interaction as a Treatment Context

Some aphasiologists [3,4] have said that treatment for people with aphasia should take place in interactional contexts. This interactional approach contrasts somewhat with structured treatment paradigms in which the clinician elicits responses to stimulate specific language processes. In our experience, people with aphasia who have participated solely in the structured type of language treatment often cannot convey functional and appropriate information when the situation demands it. Therefore, a premise of the Nebraska model is that people with aphasia need opportunities to practice communicating in a strategic and integrated manner in real-life communication contexts.

Discourse as a Treatment Context

The Nebraska group treatment model also focuses on connected discourse as an ultimate treatment goal. Ulatowska and Bond [5] suggest that the discourse level of communication should be the optimal intervention target for people with aphasia, rather than linguistic form alone. The concept of discourse implies that a communicator has a communication goal in mind and that the communication acts necessary to achieve this goal take place in a particular context. Each type of discourse (i.e., conversational, narrative, transactional, procedural, or persuasive) is governed by an implicit set of rules that dictate language content and organization (e.g., "a story has a beginning, a middle, and an end," "in a conversation you tell me stuff and ask me stuff, too"). Therefore, all communicators who engage in discourse must draw on and integrate their cognitive, pragmatic, and linguistic skills. It is not enough to retrieve words and construct sentences; communicators also must match the content of the message to their purposes, the interest and knowledge of the communication partner, and the contextual constraints of the setting. To adjust continually to the demands of co-constructing discourse, the communicator must also be able to ask questions, clarify information, and contribute equally to the evolving interaction.

Several researchers [5,6] have noted that people with aphasia often retain much of their knowledge of the structure and rules governing discourse. They also retain the desire to engage in discourse. Communicators with aphasia may participate in discourse in a limited or unsuccessful way, however, because of the constraints imposed by their disordered language system. Intervention at the discourse level can provide opportunities for people to improve the communication skills they need to interact in real-life contexts. It is our premise that choosing discourse as a treatment target allows individuals with all types and severity levels of aphasia to draw on their conceptual knowledge of the world, which builds a foundation for improving meaningful language production.

Similarly, thematicity can provide a frame for discourse-based intervention activities. Working in the frame of a theme allows participants to benefit from the gradual accumulation of context before they must deal with the complex production demands of discourse. For example, a person with aphasia may work on increasing the semantic specificity, complexity, and organization of his or her spoken output by telling a fishing story rather than repeating unrelated sentences from a stimulus list.

Scaffolding

Scaffolding refers to the process of providing cues or prompts at the leading edge of support for people who cannot yet communicate independently in complex, dynamic situations [7]. Scaffolding is particularly appropriate for people with aphasia as they search for appropriate language structures and strategies with which to communicate their ideas.

Norris and Hoffman [2] noted that clinicians have several roles when scaffolding communication in naturalistic contexts. First, the communicator must learn to attend to relevant aspects of the communication environment. Second, communication opportunities must be provided. Third, clinicians and group participants themselves must provide feedback or consequences based on how effectively the communicator influenced the listener.

Although Norris and Hoffman [2] directed their comments to therapists working with children, their framework for scaffolding is also applicable to adult language

TABLE 10-1.
Thematic Discourse Aphasia Group Therapy Model: Opening Conversation

Language Activities	Communication Goals	Scaffolding Strategies		
		Information Organization	Communication Opportunities	Consequences
Description 10–20 minutes of social conversation before thematic activity	**Attention/comprehension** Attend to others' comments or new information	Clinician directs participant to ask questions, give information, take turns	**Maximum Support** Clinician ensures that all participants have an equal number of opportunities	Clinician summarizes intent of each participant's communication act
	Social/pragmatic Ask questions Follow up Clarify Indicate others' turns Introduce topics	Gives exact verbal model and written cues as needed Provides topic		Provides feedback on adequacy of the communication efforts
Example Clinicians provide topic ideas and instruction and use props and cues to initiate conversation. Begin discussion by asking questions. Place conversational rules poster in view of all group members.	**Semantic specificity** Use specific language to convey important or new information	Uses tangible props as needed (cassette covers, newspapers, etc.) Gives some physical assistance		
	Organization of discourse Sequence information Maintain topic	Clinician uses prompts and indirect verbal models Intermittently records what participants have said Provides written or tangible topic ("You could talk about this...")	**Moderate Support** Clinician asks participants to recall who has not yet participated, then cues participants to include them ("Kris, did everyone tell us about their weekend?")	Clinician partially summarizes intent of messages and asks participants to complete summary Suggests that other participants ask for more information if unclear ("Did you get that? Ask Diane to tell us again.")
	Use of alternative communication strategies Ask questions from list Refer to stored biographical information Use breakdown strategies Introduce topic starters			
	Reading/writing Write information as needed	Clinician uses intermittent prompts Provides topic suggestions	**Minimal Support** Clinician uses minimal prompts to indicate other participants' turns	Clinician suggests that others summarize or ask for more information ("So, Harold, tell us how everyone felt.")

No Support
Participants initiate topics, questions, and new information. Participants spontaneously resolve breakdowns. Information is specific, and intent is conveyed for almost all opportunities.

intervention. In the Nebraska model, individualized levels of scaffolding (from no support to maximal support) are provided for group participants with a variety of communication challenges. General types of scaffolds include strategies to organize information from the environment, provision of adequate communication opportunities and supported communication modalities, feedback, and self-evaluation. Scaffolding strategies are reviewed in more detail under Description of Clinical Activities, below.

The components of the Nebraska scaffolded thematic discourse group treatment model are summarized in Tables 10-1 through 10-4. The model is described in more detail in the next section.

DESCRIPTION OF CLINICAL ACTIVITIES

This section illustrates the progression of therapeutic interactions within a group session. First, the four intervention phases (opening conversation, context building, language mediation, and final thematic discourse activity) are described. Then, we present techniques for scaffolding to facilitate maximal participation by group members.

Instructional Phases

Opening Conversation

Conversation is an important communication context for most adult communicators. Conversing can be an extremely challenging task for people with aphasia, however, due to the complexities of initiating topics, retrieving and encoding specific information, and channeling that information into the conversational flow at an appropriate moment. Group participants therefore are encouraged to participate in conversational interactions at every opportunity and are provided with scaffolding when necessary. For example, at the beginning of each weekly group session, the group members typically spend time conversing in the waiting area before entering the aphasia group treatment room. Clinicians passing through the waiting area frequently assist group members to engage in social automatic conversation by offering suggestions (e.g., "Sarah hasn't said hello yet. Why don't you greet her?") or direct cues (e.g., "Ask Robert, 'How are you?'") if a conversation is not already under way.

After the session officially begins in the group treatment room, clinicians provide support in a series of phases. For the first 5–10 minutes, members participate in conversation without assistance until the clinician observes that the

TABLE 10-2.
Thematic Discourse Aphasia Group Therapy Model: Context Building

Language Activities	Communication Goals	Scaffolding Strategies		
		Information Organization	Communication Opportunities	Consequences
Description 10–20 minutes of clinician-directed discussion Learning about theme and background information Small groups	**Attention/comprehension** Demonstrate comprehension of content by answering questions or using nonverbal indicators (e.g., nodding) Attend to information	**Maximum support throughout context-building activity for all participants**		
		Clinician provides visual, contextual information (tapes, pictures)	Clinician provides opportunities for all to answer questions, summarize, comment	Clinician provides feedback on adequacy of communicative efforts
	Social/pragmatic Make requests ("Stop tape.") Ask for assistance Ask for clarification Restate information	Provides prep sets, word- and sentence-level meaning cues to support text comprehension	Clinician-directed questions ("Don, what kind of music was that?")	Provides feedback on accuracy of comprehension
Example Selections of different types of music are played for all group members. Clinician posts music timeline including music types and asks participants to identify and label artists and express their likes and dislikes in music types. Participants then direct the clinician where to place music types on the timeline.	**Semantic specificity** Label music type Answer "Wh-" questions State opinion about music preference and types of music using specific terms **Organization of discourse** Summarize sentences, paragraphs, whole story Use temporal and causal connectors to organize information **Use of alternative communication strategies** Ask questions from list Refer to stored biographical information Use breakdown strategies Introduce topic starters **Reading/writing** Demonstrate reading comprehension of topic, main events, details, interrelationships, and inferential information	Provides chart with key terms and associated descriptors (music, rock and roll, jazz, etc.)		

discussion has diminished or that some members are not fully participating. During this *unsupported conversation* phase, the clinician collects data on participants' unscaffolded communication abilities via videotape recording and informal rating scales (see Figure 3-2).

In the next phase of the conversation, the *topical* phase, facilitators encourage participants to generate more specific comments by suggesting a topic. Frequently, clinicians simply point to one or more *tangible topic setters* that are prominently displayed in the room. Tangible topic setters can be newspaper headlines and photos (e.g., Olympic outcomes, a championship boxing match), bouquets of flowers from a group member's garden, used birthday candles and birthday cards, or travel photographs and postcards. In this phase of the conversation, facilitators also prompt group participants to share information about items they have brought or events that have occurred recently in their own lives. Some group participants develop a keen sense of how to include and assist other group members and are sometimes invited to lead the topical portion of the conversation.

A third phase, *supported conversation*, is initiated if some group members are not participating fully in the interaction. At this point, facilitators might provide verbal, gestural, and contextual cues at a variety of scaffolding levels to encourage group members to initiate questions or provide information. Table 10-5 gives an example of a scaffolded group conversation involving a 40-year-old man with profound expressive aphasia.

In contrast to the spontaneously evolving group conversation, the next three phases of group therapy sessions typically center on a thematic discourse activity selected by group members or clinicians in advance. Some thematic discourse topics used in the Nebraska group therapy program pertained to world or local community events with a shared importance to group members (e.g., writing a letter to the Nebraska football coach after the team won the national championship; debating and critiquing Nancy Kerrigan's and Tonya Harding's skating performances in the 1994 Olympics). Other topics were daily life events and communication challenges (e.g., practicing how to ask for a specific haircut or procedure at the beauty salon,

TABLE 10-3.
Thematic Discourse Aphasia Group Therapy Model: Language Mediation

Language Activities	Communication Goals	Scaffolding Strategies		
		Information Organization	*Communication Opportunities*	*Consequences*
Description	**Attention/comprehension**	Clinician organizes key elements of chart and discourse activity (see Figure 10-2) Supplements written words with pictures Provides direct verbal model as needed	**Maximum Support**	Clinician interprets, affirms, or acknowledges all communication efforts Provides feedback on adequacy of message Requests repairs Requests additional information or expansions
Clinician-facilitated 45-minute small-group activity in which clients map language onto ideas that they will ultimately communicate in a discourse activity	Attend to and comprehend information presented by others		Clinician directs participants to request opinions of others ("Ask Joe what he thinks of rock music.") Ensures all participants have an equal number of turns Provides cues as needed (semantic, phonemic, sentence completion)	
Interactive information-sharing	**Social/pragmatic** Provide information Ask questions of others, take turns ("What do you think?") Comment ("Music was OK.") Ask follow-up questions ("Why?") Clarify			
Example	**Semantic specificity**	Same as maximum support Clinician also encourages participants to add information and use other descriptors	**Moderate Support**	Clinician prompts participants to comment on information that has been shared ("Tell Sam whether you agree or not.")
Participants take turns reading and making choices on a survey sheet. Sentence starter phrases and written choices are included on the survey for participants with decreased ability to generate language. Participants are encouraged to add other comments or information and to state opinions. Rating scale included on chart to facilitate commenting and opinion sharing. Music selections are reviewed as needed.	Use specific descriptors (classic, country, rock, rap) Use specific nouns (tape, radio, compact disc) Use connected semantic relations ("I like rock music.")		Clinician prompts others to say "What do you think?" or "Your turn."	
	Organization of discourse Connect information in a logical descriptive sequence ("I like rock music; my favorite singer is _____. I listen to music on tapes.") Use causal connectors to mark opinions ("I like my music 'cause it sounds good.")	Clinician prompts participants to complete connected discourse activity without reading verbatim from chart or survey sheets	**Minimal Support** Clinician occasionally prompts participants to ask questions of others	Clinician prompts participants to comment or respond to information that has been shared using open-ended prompts ("And you feel...")
	Use of alternative communication strategies Refer others to prewritten information Draw or write to add information Gesture (thumbs up = good)		**No Support**	
	Reading/writing Copy selected words into sentence formats Read key words and sentences aloud	Participants practice sharing opinions and summarizing information with peers. Independently use written or visual references as needed. Give feedback to each other regarding the adequacy of the message.		

ordering Girl Scout cookies from a neighborhood girl, asking their kids to clean up their rooms). Some activities focused on reminiscing. Still other activities allowed group members to share expertise in an area such as golfing, gardening, or changing a tire on a car.

To prepare group members for maximal participation in a discourse activity, group members then engage in context building, language mediation, and final discourse performance.

Context Building
In this phase of the thematic discourse activity, the clinician first prepares the room with *visual contextual cues*. For example, when group members discussed their favorite type of music, pictures of musicians, sheet music, cassette covers,

and signs depicting the topic of music provided visual context. The clinician may then ask general questions about music preferences, such as "Do any of you listen to music?" Additional opportunities for taking turns are signaled with cues such as, "Margaret, can you find out?" The clinician also provides opportunities for elaboration, as appropriate. To tap into participants' recollections of personal experiences or associations with the theme, the clinician then asks personal experience questions, such as, "Who were your favorite musical stars when you were a kid?"

Next, to promote language comprehension and recall of episodic information without taxing expressive language abilities, the clinicians usually attempt to provide more *active participation experiences* for group participants. During the music preference activity, people were asked to

TABLE 10-4.
Thematic Discourse Aphasia Group Therapy Model: Final Discourse Activity

		Scaffolding Strategies		
Language Activities	*Communication Goals*	*Information Organization*	*Communication Opportunities*	*Consequences*
Description Clinicians and all participants return to large-group format. Each participant must organize information and communicate it in a goal-directed manner to the group. Discourse activities can include description or story-telling, transactions, procedural or instructional descriptions, persuasion or debate **Example** Participants inform others of their music preferences. They indicate where that style of music is located on the timeline. Clinicians encourage some participants to increase the complexity of their discourse by adding information or expanding the semantic or grammatic complexity of their utterances. Participants then restate music preference. Clinicians facilitate group inferential thinking or predictions in a brief question-and-answer exchange at end of session ("Do you think you would buy music the next time you shop? Could you ask a store clerk for new country music hits?")	**Attention/comprehension** Listen and comprehend other participants' discourse Answer questions pertaining to the topic or information shared by others Add new, related information **Social/pragmatic** Provide information Ask questions of others, take turns ("What do you think?") Comment ("Music was OK.") Ask follow-up questions ("Why?") Clarify Less scaffolding **Semantic specificity** Use specific descriptors (classic, country, rock, rap) Use specific nouns (tape, radio, compact disc) Use connected semantic relations ("I like rock music.") Less scaffolding **Organization of discourse** Connect information in a logical descriptive sequence ("I like rock music; my favorite singer is ____. I listen to music on tapes.") Use casual connectors to mark opinions ("I like my music 'cause it sounds good.") Less scaffolding **Use of alternative communication strategies** Refer others to prewritten information Draw or write to add information Gesture (thumbs up = good) Reading/writing Read notes or worksheets silently or aloud when information review is necessary Writing used to organize thoughts or resolve communication breakdowns Note: Participants are asked to evaluate their performance on these objectives at the end of the discourse activity (e.g., "How did you do? Show us on this scale.")	Clinician organizes key elements of chart and discourse activity (see attached). Supplements written words with pictures Provides direct verbal model as needed	**Maximum Support** Clinician directs participants to request opinions of others ("Ask Joe what he thinks of rock music.") Ensures all participants have an equal number of turns Provides cues as needed (semantic, phonemic, sentence completion)	Clinician interprets, affirms, or acknowledges all communication efforts Provides feedback on adequacy of message Requests repairs Requests additional information or expansions
		Same as maximum support Clinician encourages participants to add information and use other descriptors	**Moderate Support** Clinician prompts others to say "What do you think?" or "Your turn."	Clinician prompts participants to comment on information that has been shared
		Clinician prompts participants to complete connected discourse activity without reading verbatim from chart or survey sheets	**Minimal Support** Clinician occasionally prompts participants to ask questions of others	Clinician prompts participants to comment or respond to information that has been shared

No Support
Participant describes his or her music preference with specificity, clarity, accuracy of relationships and reference; uses a logical organizational schema or order; embellishes basic information using a variety of rich semantic descriptions; supports opinion by incorporating previously stated facts into causal statements; incorporates more than one point of view and relates own view to views of others; asks questions of others at end of own turn.

TABLE 10-5.
Sample Scaffolded Conversation Involving a Man with Severe Expressive Aphasia and Other Group Participants

Context: Jerry's daughter was married before the last group meeting. His wife helped him to bring a variety of objects (a wedding invitation, a package of rice, and a snapshot of Jerry with his daughter in her bridal gown) to "tell" other group members about the wedding.

Supported group conversation:

Clinician: "Well, we all know that Jerry had a big event take place in his life last week . . ." [opportunity cue: pause]

Jerry: [No communication attempt]

Clinician: "Why don't you show them?" [opportunity cue: indicates that Jerry should retrieve items related to the wedding]

Jerry: [Pulls out photos, etc., and shows them to group members; they begin to comment and ask questions.]

Clinician: "Listen to what Jerry says about his daughter. He's going to tell you that his daughter got . . ." [opportunity cues: expectant pause and rising intonation]

Jerry: "Married."

Clinician: "Right, Jerry. However, I don't think everyone heard you. You said your daughter got . . ." [opportunity cue pause]

Jerry: "Married."

Clinician: "Wow, I bet you were a proud dad. Why doesn't someone find out more information about the wedding . . ." [opportunity cue: gestures to other group members]

Gracie: "Sue . . . sue . . ." [points to her dress]

Clinician: "Sounds like Gracie wants to know what her dress was like, right?" [feedback, interpretation]

Gracie: [Nods]

Clinician: [Pauses, no response from Jerry, generates written choices] "Was the dress . . ."
• Fancy, lots of lace
• Simple, elegant

Jerry: [Points to "simple, elegant"]

Clinician: [Circles choice; feedback: ask another group member to confirm]

Mary: "Oh, a simple dress."

Ben: "Music, music?" [gestures like an orchestra conductor]

Clinician: "Jerry, I think Ben wants to know, 'Did you have music?'"

Jerry: "Yes."

Mary: "What . . . uh . . . what kind of music, Jerry?"

Jerry: [Gestures with one hand like he's playing a violin with a bow]

Mary: "I don't understand." [feedback]

Clinician: "Jerry, did you have . . ." [writes choices]
• Organ music
• Violin music
• Flutes

Jerry: [Points to violins]

Mary: "Oh, violins . . . that's nice.

Ben: "That's nice . . . money . . . money?"

Clinician: [Generates written augmented input for Bob: "Money"]

Bob: "Money . . . yes, lots of money."

Mary: "Did you . . . uh . . . lots of money . . . did it cost lots of money?"

Jerry: [Shakes hand vaguely]

Clinician: [Generates a graphic rating scale]

Cheap   Expensive
<———/———/———/———>
1   2   3   4   5

Jerry: [Points to 5, shakes head]

Mary: "Oh, it was really expensive. My daughter's, too!" [laughs]

---

match different musical styles and artists (e.g., Elvis, rock and roll, rap) to different decades printed on a large graphic timeline (Figure 10-1). Some people, particularly those who could not communicate verbally, chose to approach the timeline and physically attach pictures to the chart. Others communicated their ideas verbally ("Elvis, yeah, woo woo"). Another active participation experience for this activity involved listening to brief segments of music selections and commenting in basic terms (e.g., gesturing thumbs up or thumbs down; "No way") about their preferences or reactions to the music.

Other context-building activities have included reading simplified articles about a topic, watching clinicians role-play a community transaction (e.g., buying a lottery ticket) and critiquing their performances, choosing favorite recipes from a cookbook before a discussion of cooking, viewing a videotaped segment of the Olympics, selecting favorite flowers from gardening catalogs, reviewing props and materials used in a particular situation (e.g., golfing items), or sequencing the steps to a procedural activity (e.g., how to exercise). On completion of this phase of the discourse activity, participants should demonstrate awareness and recognition of the tasks, topics, or communication challenges that are about to be addressed in more detail in the next phases.

Language Mediation

In this clinician-facilitated phase, communicators work in small groups. The goal of this phase is to map language onto ideas that are ultimately communicated in the final discourse activity. Using a survey or worksheet as a starting point, participants are encouraged to narrate, make comments, state opinions, or practice scripts. Clinicians also assist people to prepare communication strategies for the final discourse activity. For example, when planning for the music debate, the clinicians encouraged group members to think of people in the large group who would potentially disagree with their opinion. In other situations, clinicians coach participants to think of nonverbal communication strategies, such as pantomiming or using their communication notebooks, if they have been unable to produce target language structures during language mediation.

For example, to prepare for the debate about music preferences, group participants first completed a survey sheet about their own musical likes and dislikes with clinician assistance as needed. For participants with limited generative language, sentence starter phrases and written choices were included. Open-ended statements or suggestions were provided for participants with good verbal expression skills (Figure 10-2). Rating scales facilitated commenting and opinion sharing. The group members then practiced narrating their musical preferences and debating their choices with others.

Other examples of language mediation activities include practicing scripts to buy a lottery ticket, reviewing the steps to an exercise program in preparation for teaching others an exercise routine, following a graphic outline or flow chart to tell a story, constructing a story page for a personal reminiscence book, or reciting the steps of a recipe using cooking utensil props and an enlarged recipe card.

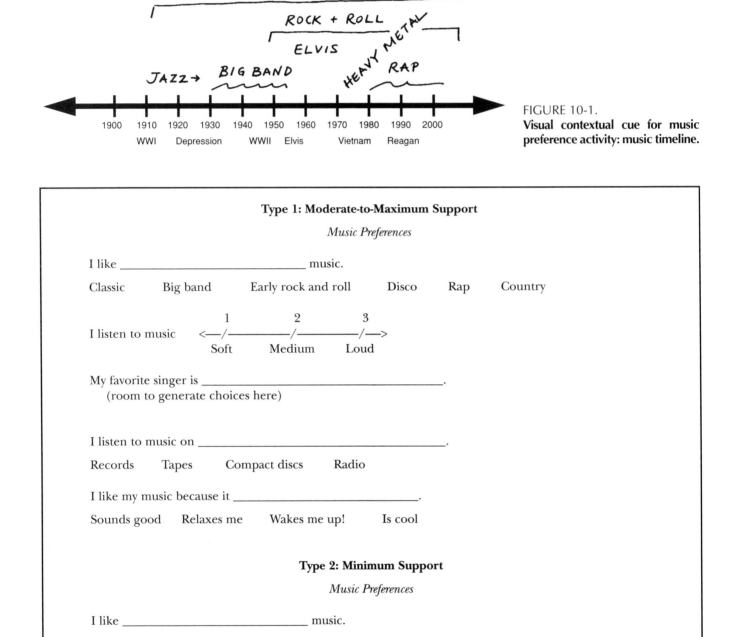

FIGURE 10-1.
Visual contextual cue for music preference activity: music timeline.

FIGURE 10-2.
Sample language mediation worksheets across scaffolding levels.

TABLE 10-6.
Final Discourse Activity: Teaching Group Members How to Play Golf

Clinician:	"OK, next Jerry and Ben are going to teach us about a sport they love."
Ben:	"Golf."
Jerry:	[Picks up club] "Hit. Golf."
Ben:	"Ball [picks up ball], glove, cub . . . no, club, shoes, shorts, tee [shows tee]."
Clinician:	"So, that looks like we'd need some . . ."
Ben:	"Equipment."
Clinician:	"So then . . ."
Ben:	"Ball . . . [places ball on tee] watch."
Jerry:	[Gets club, holds it in swinging position]
Ben:	"No, no. [repositions club] Two hands."
Jerry:	[Grins] "Two hands."
Clinician:	"And now you . . ."
Ben and Jerry:	"Swing." [swings club]
Group member:	"Going, going, gone!"

Final Discourse "Performance"

After language mediation, group participants return to the large group for the final discourse activity. This final "performance" provides another opportunity for group members to target their communication goals, this time in a more dynamic and interactive context. In this phase, group members have described their music preferences, argued about skating routines, taught each other how to bake cakes or play golf, and ordered cookies from a clinician posing as a Girl Scout. Each communicator has an initial opportunity to share ideas and information without interruption. However, interactions quickly expand in a unique and dynamic manner, as all participants are encouraged to add information, comment, argue, or ask questions of their peers. When needed, clinicians stimulate the interaction by providing cues and prompts for speakers and their partners.

For an illustration of a final procedural discourse session, see Table 10-6 for an example of a discourse activity in which two men, one with severe and one with moderate aphasia, teach the rest of the group how to golf.

Specific Scaffolding Strategies

In each session, some participants require assistance to participate maximally in the discourse activities. Three types of supports are used: environmental organization, communication opportunities, and feedback or consequences. First, to organize the environment for participants, a variety of visual contextual cues are used, including tangible or pictorial topic setters, spontaneously generated flow charts or outlines of possible ways to extend conversational topics, timelines and story charts, charts depicting conversational reminders, props for discourse activities, simplified or enlarged articles from magazines and newspapers, and written scripts for rehearsal of role-plays. To supplement the auditory comprehension of some people, *augmented input* [8], or the provision of written key words during an evolving interaction, is used as needed. Clinicians also use verbal and nonverbal *interac-*

tional guide cues, such as pointing to the individual who is talking, to assist some participants to follow the interactional flow.

To ensure that all participants have enough opportunities to participate in conversation or thematic discourse activities, a hierarchy of cues is used. Typically, facilitators begin with the least restrictive cue, such as pausing or encouraging other participants to allow enough time for a fellow group member to communicate. If this level of cueing is insufficient, the clinicians might offer suggestions about a possible topic ("Can you tell us about your weekend?"), strategy ("Can you show us in your book?"), or a potential recipient of a communication message (e.g., "We haven't heard from John. Why don't you ask him?"). When participants supply partial messages or offer bits of information that are not organized in a temporal or relational flow, *cohesive tie cues* (e.g., "and," "then") are sometimes offered. Facilitators might also summarize information that has been discussed or restate messages that have been partially communicated so that the individual can more efficiently formulate the remainder of the message. Written choices are offered to people who cannot communicate information verbally. This strategy [8] allows people with severe expressive communication challenges to offer novel information by pointing to one of a set of written words that are possible answers to conversational questions. Using this technique, communicators can also share opinions or qualitative responses by pointing to marks on a rating scale (see the written choice and rating scale examples in Table 10-5). *Language cues* (e.g., opposites, sentence completion, phonemic) are offered when an individual clearly knows what he or she wants to say but cannot successfully retrieve the target words using any other strategy. *Repetition cues* and *verbal models* are offered when an individual has no other means of producing the language form. These levels of cueing (language cues, verbal models, and repetition) are used sparingly for two reasons: They promote cue dependence, and they violate principles of communicative sincerity (i.e., clinicians already know the communicator's message before delivering the cue). Finally, facilitators sometimes provide physical assistance so that group members can open pages in their communication notebook, gesture, or indicate another's turn.

To ensure that some people with limited verbal expression skills have opportunities to access semantically specific information, a variety of augmentative communication strategies are sometimes used. Some people use *stored information notebooks* to communicate about their background, family, typical weekend events, recent news, common question forms, or other predictable items of information. When appropriate, communicators obtain scripts for upcoming transactions that were previously stored in the notebook. Other people communicate unique information with strategies such as writing on a tablet, pointing to locations on a map, or pointing to the first letter of a key word on an alphabet card. During group sessions, maps, calendars, paper, pens, and alphabet cards are continuously available to support these types of spontaneous, augmented communication acts.

TABLE 10-7.
Sample Opportunity Cues across Scaffolding Levels

Minimal cues:
  (a) "Looks like Jerry is refreshed; I wonder if he had an interesting weekend?"
  (b) "This looks interesting." [facilitator points to newspaper article]
  (c) "And . . . ?" [cue to elaborate]
  (d) [Long pause to provide time for individual to formulate answer]
Moderate cues:
  (a) "Looks like Jerry is refreshed; I wonder if he had an interesting weekend?" [point to group member and then to adjacent member] "Can you find out?"
  (b) "Can you tell us in another way?"
  (c) "Can you tell us what you did?"
Maximal cues:
  (a) "Ask Mary, 'Who [did you go with]?' "
  (b) "Show Ben where you went—look at the green pages in your notebook."
  (c) Written choices: "Did you go to the cabin or stay at home this weekend?" [Facilitator writes "cabin" and "home" simultaneously and indicates communicator should point to the answer]

Some other people have used simple *voice output communication aids (VOCAs)* with one to eight message-selection spaces for participation in certain communication activities. For example, one individual used an eight-message digitized VOCA to participate in the opening conversational sequence until his natural speech and gestures evolved to support his participation. Other people have used portable VOCAs for brief periods to participate partially in community role-plays.

We found that it was possible to adapt most activities to meet the unique needs of people with long-term aphasia, even when groups were mixed with regard to severity levels. This sometimes required the clinician to provide more overt cues to the individual with moderate-to-severe receptive and expressive aphasia (e.g., "John, why don't you ask Eva, 'How was your weekend?' Can you use your notebook?"). In contrast, for people with relatively strong verbal expression skills but poor discourse organization, the clinician may be able to assist by writing out the cue "Friday-Saturday-Sunday," and then asking the individual, "I wonder what Edward did this weekend?" Table 10-7 provides additional examples of how cues can be modified according to the level of scaffolding needed by the person with aphasia.

Facilitators also try to provide feedback as well as frequent opportunities for participants to self-evaluate their communication. In conversation, group members often are asked to evaluate message adequacy and naturalness on a turn-by-turn basis (e.g., "Ben, do you think Carrie understood that? How else could you explain your opinion?"). Other group members are frequently encouraged to respond, comment, or request message repairs. During role-plays and "rehearsals" for the final discourse activity, people sometimes assess how they communicated by completing a simple questionnaire (Figure 10-3). At other times, group members watch and verbally critique a videotape of their performance. Throughout the semester, group participants also are encouraged to share their per-

ceptions of how well they communicated in similar situations at home or in the community.

A corollary principle of scaffolding used in the Nebraska thematic discourse model is the provision of *multiple opportunities* for participants to manipulate information in meaningful contexts. People with impaired language systems may need more than one opportunity to comprehend, connect, and use language forms to accomplish communication goals as independently as possible. To this end, group participants receive repeated opportunities to participate in conversational discourse, to demonstrate comprehension during context building, to map language forms onto ideas during language mediation, and to role-play and rehearse during the final discourse phase of the session.

ADDITIONAL PROGRAM INFORMATION

Entry and Discharge Criteria

People with all types of aphasia profiles, levels of severity (mild to profound), ages, and backgrounds were eligible to participate in the University of Nebraska–Lincoln adult aphasia group treatment program. Primary referral sources included a local rehabilitation hospital, the local stroke support group, family members, the university community, and private practitioners in the area. In general, people continued participating in the program under three conditions: (1) continued quantitative and qualitative changes in their functional communication ability; (2) presence of unmet communication needs at home, work, or in the community; and (3) continued motivation to attend. Some people periodically "raised the yardstick" and identified areas (e.g., public speaking, reading, writing) in which they wanted to further improve their communication skills. Other criteria included regular attendance, adequate health and endurance to participate in the treatment session, and scheduling and transportation logistics.

Length and Frequency of Group Sessions

Typically, weekly group sessions lasted 90 minutes. Six to 10 people with aphasia participated in each group session. Group treatment was often supplemented with individual treatment sessions, depending on client need and logistics.

Assessment

We obtained communication profiles of group members soon after their enrollment in group therapy for two purposes: to provide student clinicians with information about the nature of group members' speech, language, and communication skills and to obtain some benchmarks for outcome evaluation. Results of testing were not used to

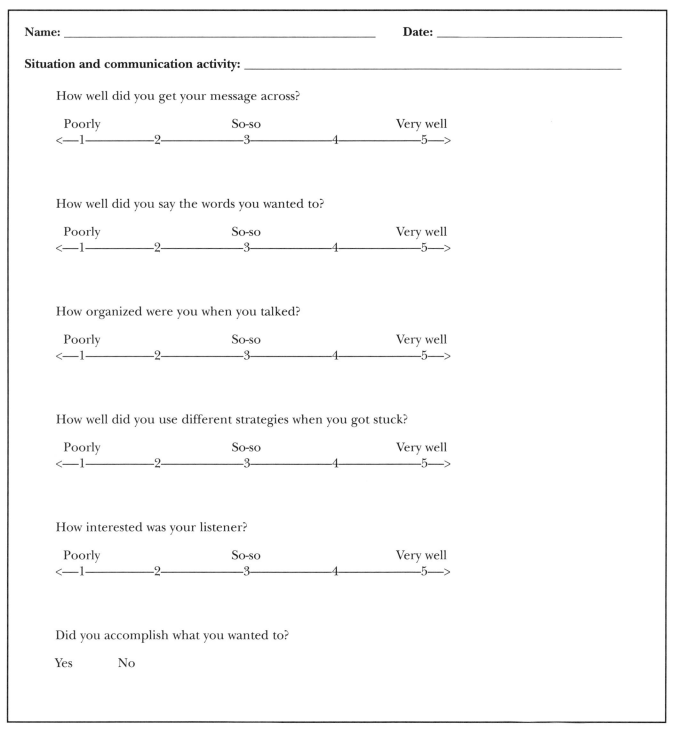

FIGURE 10-3.
Group participant discourse evaluation tool. (Courtesy of Kathryn L. Garrett and Gayle J. Ellis; used with permission.)

determine candidacy for group treatment. As a general guideline, the following parameters were assessed via formal and informal measures: (1) language ability (expressive, receptive, reading, writing), (2) motor speech and apraxia, (3) cognitive skills, (4) interaction skills, and (5) functional measures of communicative competence. Formal assessment information was typically obtained in individual treatment sessions or from reports from the person's most recent rehabilitation program. In addition, the communicators and their significant communication partners sometimes completed informal rating scales to assess functional communication competence and status of communication needs.

Staffing

The group therapy program was staffed and supervised by two university clinical supervisors. Two to five student clinicians were assigned to the adult aphasia treatment group each semester; group clinicians also typically worked on an individual basis with at least one of the group members. Initially, group supervisors served as primary facilitators in the group activities, thereby providing a model for student clinicians. As the semester progressed, students assumed primary responsibility for planning and facilitating activities but continued to meet weekly with supervisors to refine their plans and discuss scaffolding strategies. In most sessions, spouses or other communication partners chose to observe group activities from an observation room, where they talked with each other about the challenges associated with stroke and aphasia. As the semester progressed, supervisors observed activities from this observation room as well. They could then discuss communication and life adjustment issues with family members and gather information about the communication abilities of group members in outside situations.

Treatment Goals

Formal treatment goals and objectives were identified for all clients who participated in group therapy. Many of the specific skills targeted in group (attention and comprehension, semantic specificity, organization of discourse, pragmatics, use of alternative communication strategies, and reading comprehension and writing) were also included in individual treatment plans.

Documentation of Progress

In general, progress was tracked by (1) obtaining data on completion of specific objectives, (2) periodically videotaping sessions and re-rating interaction skills with the Informal Discourse Rating Scale (see Figure 3-2), (3) interviewing participants and family members to determine if communication needs were met or if they perceived qualitative differences in their lives, and (4) intermittently readministering formal tests.

Reimbursement Issues

When group participants first enrolled in the therapy program, every effort was made to obtain third-party payer funding for them. We obtained complete insurance or vocational rehabilitation funding for approximately 10% of the participants and partial funding (e.g., coverage for 60 consecutive calendar days) for another 15%. Medicaid funding was available for approximately 25% of participants, although reimbursement rates were minimal and did not cover costs. Medicare reimbursement efforts for participants older than 65 years of age were largely unsuccessful. Clients without third-party payer sources were asked to contribute financially to the group according to a sliding-scale fee schedule based on a minimum fee of $5 per session. Financial support from local civic groups (e.g., Sertoma, Jaycees) also generated tuition scholarships for some people. Because we served as a training institution for graduate students, who supplied the program with tuition money, the university assumed many of the overhead costs associated with providing a group therapy program (e.g., supervisor salaries, building costs).

SUMMARY

The Nebraska model of group therapy was developed to meet the communication challenges of people with long-term aphasia. It is our continued belief that a focus on discourse is a natural way to extend intervention and improve overall communication competence. The use of meaningful thematic activities facilitated successful interactions in a wider variety of communication environments and with a greater number of communication partners than were available in individual treatment. The instructional components of our group model also allowed student clinicians to understand how to scaffold people with aphasia to participate to their fullest in interactional discourse.

Throughout the 4 years in which the Nebraska group model functioned, group participants and their significant communication partners frequently commented that the sessions were functional, meaningful, and helped them achieve their goal of becoming more competent communicators. To illustrate, during the 1996 presidential election, voting emerged as a natural theme. After participating in conversations and discourse activities about the election for several weeks, one 47-year-old woman with mild aphasia revealed that for the first time since her stroke, she had voted on her own. In our current work environments, we will focus on measuring outcomes and validating the impact of the scaffolded thematic discourse approach to group treatment on the communication of adults with long-term aphasia.

REFERENCES

1. Garrett K, Ellis G. Miniseminar: group therapy for persons with long-term aphasia: scaffolded language activities. Presented at the Annual American Speech-Language Association Convention, New Orleans, LA, November, 1994.
2. Norris JA, Hoffman P. Language intervention within naturalistic environments. Lang Speech Hear Serv Sch 1990;21:72–84.
3. Bloom L. A rationale for group treatment of aphasic patients. J Speech Hear Disord 1962;27:11–16.
4. Aten J, Caligiuri M, Holland A. The efficacy of functional communication therapy for chronic aphasic patients. J Speech Hear Disord 1982;47:93–96.
5. Ulatowska H, Bond S. Aphasia: Discourse considerations. Top Lang Disord 1983;3:21–34.
6. Holland A. Observing functional communication in aphasic adults. J Speech Hear Disord 1977;47:50–56.
7. Mastergeorge A, Olswang L, Bain B. Socio-cultural history and context in intervention: rethinking dynamic approaches. A seminar presented at the Annual American Speech-Language-Hearing Association Convention, Boston, MA, November, 1997.
8. Garrett KL, Beukelman DR. Severe Aphasia. In KM Yorkston (ed), Augmentative Communication in the Medical Setting. Tucson, AZ: Communication Skill Builders, 1992;245–321.

Part Three: Volunteer-Facilitated Groups

CHAPTER ELEVEN

Groups in the Introductory Program at the Pat Arato Aphasia Centre

Aura Kagan and
Rochelle Cohen-Schneider

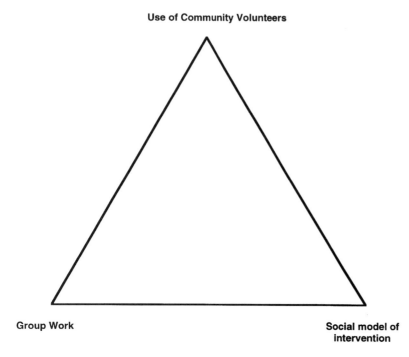

Use of Community Volunteers

Group Work

Social model of intervention

FIGURE 11-1.
Key elements of service delivery at the Pat Arato Aphasia Centre.

Pat Arato's husband had a stroke with accompanying aphasia at a young age. After his discharge from therapy, she became aware of the critical need for some kind of ongoing support for him and others in the same position. In 1979, she founded the Aphasia Centre–North York, which has recently been renamed the Pat Arato Aphasia Centre* in her honor.

Three factors characterize the approach to service delivery used at the center (Figure 11-1). The first two, the participation of community volunteers and the use of groups, have been constants since the founding of the Centre. The third component, the philosophic underpinning, has evolved to what can be described as a social model based on increasing the communicative access of aphasic adults to meaningful participation in everyday life [1–3].

The Centre runs many and varied groups within different programs. Volunteer-led conversation groups for our aphasic members have historically distinguished the Centre's approach.

By definition, conversation involves partnerships, and we therefore spend a large proportion of our time and energy on the training and supervision of volunteer conversation partners for our aphasic members. Specifically, they are given training in the use of the resources and techniques of Supported Conversation for Adults with Aphasia (SCA) [1,2]. Volunteers are taught techniques that enable them to (1) acknowledge and (2) reveal the inherent competence of adults with aphasia within the

framework of natural adult conversation. When we use the term *conversational support*, we mean the use of these techniques and resource materials. Most of our volunteers are students who want to apply to speech-language pathology departments at various universities. Other volunteers come from a range of backgrounds. The Centre recruits volunteers through a public volunteer agency and via radio, television, presentations, and notices in appropriate public venues.

The Centre has developed a sophisticated Introductory Program that is the gateway to the Centre's services. It is offered to the person with aphasia and to family members or friends, preparing them for participation in our Community Aphasia Program (CAP) and other programs outside the Centre. Groups in the Introductory Program form the subject matter of this chapter. These groups are also volunteer-run and conversation-based, but they have a formal psychoeducational agenda in addition to the focus on free-flowing natural conversation.

Groups available in the CAP include special-interest or activity groups such as cooking or music, skill-building groups focusing on reading and writing, peer-training groups, family support and education groups, and, of course, generic conversation groups (Figure 11-2). Most groups are facilitated by volunteers, but some, such as the family support and education groups, are run by professional social workers and speech-language pathology staff.

All groups include opportunities for conversation, but in our generic conversation groups, conversation itself is the activity. When we use the phrase "opportunity for genuine conversation," we refer to an emphasis on forgetting about the communication problem and concentrating on the conversational interaction and content for its own sake. We focus on what aphasic group members and vol-

*The Pat Arato Aphasia Centre, 53 The Links Road, North York, Ontario, Canada, M2P 1T7; Web site: http://www.aphasia.on.ca; e-mail: aphasia@ibm.net.

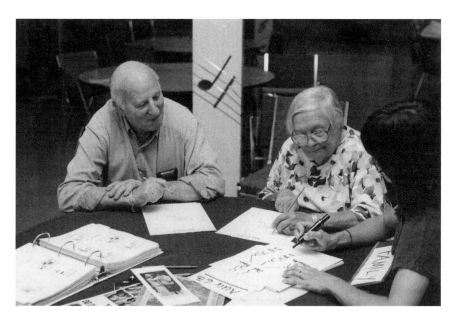

FIGURE 11-2.
Group session incorporating Supported Conversation for Adults with Aphasia.

unteer facilitators achieve together rather than on independent transmission of information.* In keeping with the "social approach" to aphasia [4,5], success in this area requires that volunteers let go of the "fixer" role. Although our Introductory Program groups have a psychosocial and psychoeducational agenda, staff and volunteers put considerable effort into ensuring that a large proportion of time is spent on providing genuine conversational opportunities.

To cope with a large demand for service and limited staff resources, the Centre currently operates programs in three 4-month terms per year. Service is provided for more than 300 people with aphasia (mostly post-stroke) and their families during any one term, with the help of approximately 100 volunteers. Such service includes work during the intake stage, requests for help, and direct service to our aphasic members and their families. Volunteers put in approximately 16,000 hours of work each year, the bulk of which is working directly with aphasic people, largely within group settings. The Centre employs a full-time coordinator of volunteers who is responsible for recruitment, administration, support, and supervision in areas that do not require professional expertise. Other staff include the executive director, an office manager, three full-time equivalent speech-language pathology positions divided among five staff members, and two part-time social workers sharing less than one position.

Before moving on to a detailed description of the groups in our Introductory Program, we outline the typi-

cal path that a potential applicant with aphasia and his family follows from the time of referral.

Let us assume that a man with aphasia (John) is referred to the Centre in term 1. A member of the professional staff makes a follow-up telephone call. Some counseling and information is given at this point, and John and his family are offered an introductory visit by a team made up of a speech-language pathologist and a social worker. The visit takes place in term 2. If John is appropriate for the program and he chooses to attend, he and his family are offered a place in our 12-week Introductory Program in term 3. After participation in the Introductory Program, John can choose to join the CAP, where there is a choice of activities each term. New members are encouraged to join generic conversation groups first, to solidify gains made in the Introductory Program. As with any community center, people can choose whether to sign up for any particular session.

ENTRY CRITERIA

Applicants to the Centre are usually referred by speech-language pathologists. They are required to fill out a standard referral form and attach reports. Because our staff resources are limited, we find it useful to collect clinical information during the acute and rehabilitation phase. On occasion, referrals are made by other health care professionals. To activate the referral and have a file opened, we ask for access to the report of the last speech-language pathologist consulted. We assist applicants who have not had a speech-language pathology assessment.

To qualify for a place in the Introductory Program, applicants must meet the following criteria:

- Aphasia is the predominant problem; concomitant disorders (e.g., apraxia, dysarthria, or cognitive-communicative deficits) are less prominent than the aphasia.

---

*At the Centre, work on functional communication, or what we term *communication effectiveness training,* does form part of our activities but is differentiated from the offering of opportunities for natural conversation. Communication effectiveness training is also done in a group format.

- They can sustain participation in a group meeting that lasts for 1.5 hours.
- They do not have inappropriate behavior (e.g., violent outbursts or wandering).
- They do not have any degenerative condition other than progressive aphasia. (We are currently doing pilot work to see whether we can meet the needs of this population.)
- Ideally, they are at least 10 months to 1 year post-onset when entering the program. The Introductory Program is designed specifically for clients who are beginning to face the chronicity of their aphasia.

Our referral agents do not necessarily refer every aphasic client on their caseloads. There are a number of reasons for this:

- Clients do not live close enough to attend.
- Clients may not enjoy a group setting.
- Clients may speak a language other than English and may not wish to participate in programming in English.
- The speech-language pathologist may deem a candidate unsuitable. Clients at either end of the severity continuum may be excluded.

We receive approximately 10 referrals each month. Challenges facing us include the fact that we rely on speech-language pathologists in the acute and rehabilitation phase to encourage clients to participate in the Centre's programs. To do this, clinicians need to understand and support the Centre's philosophy and be kept up to date with policy and programming changes. We hold annual meetings to do this. Informal, ongoing links are maintained by the program staff.

ASSESSMENT

The social worker initiates the assessment process with a telephone call to the applicant or a family member, depending on the circumstances. In this first conversation, we gain information about the applicant's emotional status and knowledge of aphasia. An appointment is set up for an introductory visit with a staff team comprised of a social worker and a speech-language pathologist. Referrals for additional or alternative services may also be made at this stage, depending on the applicant's needs.

The introductory visit is conducted in the applicant's home, if possible. In some instances, due to limited staff resources, visits may need to be done at the Centre. Applicants with severe aphasia have priority for a home visit. If the visit is held at the Centre, applicants are asked to bring in photographs and any artifacts that tell us more about who they are. The staff team first meets with the applicant and his family together. Using a pictographic assessment–interview guide, the speech-language pathologist begins chatting with the aphasic applicant, covering topics such as what has happened to him or her. Within a short time, the speech-language pathologist

forms an idea of whether or not they are able to exchange information and use conversational supports, such as pictographic resource material and written keywords. In almost all cases, even where aphasia is described as global, we do manage to get some conversation going and are then able to split the interview. The social worker chats with the family member, and the speech-language pathologist continues with the aphasic applicant. The content of the interviews is the same; the only difference is the conversational support offered to the aphasic individual. Everyone comes together for a final summary of what has been learned. The Introductory Program is described, and the applicant decides whether he or she is interested in enrolling. The applicant has an opportunity to discuss personal goals and expectations using a pictographic representation of the "downward fall" after the stroke and the potential for "steps forward."

The team writes a report immediately after the visit. The pictographic interview document, with its clear indications of what has changed and what is of current concern, forms an integral part of record-keeping. Notes are written in a format that is accessible to volunteers, who are required to sign confidentiality contracts before each program. Information regarded as too personal or not necessary for volunteers to know is put into our regular member files, which are confidential to professional staff.

Information gained from the introductory visit is used in forming groups for the 12-week Introductory Program. Grouping is based on severity of aphasia, personality, interests, and goals. This information is also taken into account when assigning volunteers to each group. In the two preparatory meetings before each Introductory Program begins, a staff person from the introductory visit team gives volunteers in-depth information about incoming members, concentrating particularly on getting a sense of the people behind the disorder. Photographs taken at the introductory visit are shown to connect further the volunteers to their group members.

TREATMENT GOALS PROGRAM

According to our mission statement, "The Introductory Program provides a peer-group framework for conversations about aphasia in relation to future plans for members with aphasia and their families."

Specific goals and objectives are as follows:

- To provide a supportive social environment for new aphasic members and their families
- To work on techniques for improving communicative effectiveness
- To provide a forum for conversation about aphasia from various angles: individual stories of "what happened," education about aphasia, the current reality of living with aphasia, and opportunities for the future

- To provide a bridge to the CAP for those planning to continue their association with the Centre
- To introduce concrete ideas about "the next step" (including ideas for participation in family, in the Centre community, and in other community activities)
- To provide concurrent support and education for families and friends of our aphasic members

In this context, goals are set for individual group participants, building on the conversation that was started at the introductory visit. Goal setting is an underlying theme of the Introductory Program. This allows members to look forward, plan, and take some control of, and responsibility for, their future.

PROGRAM DOCUMENTATION

Informal documentation of members' progress takes place in the weekly meetings held before and after each group session. Volunteers report on events in their group, share experiences, and ask for help with challenging group members or situations. Concerns are noted by program staff and dealt with either in the volunteer meeting or in individual meetings with the volunteer, if necessary. We have seen a positive change in the depth of discussion in our volunteer meetings since we have increased our investment of time in the intake process. We attribute this to the availability of improved background information about the members, including knowledge of personal priorities and goals, as well as better understanding of family dynamics.

Formal clinical documentation begins with notes on the goals articulated verbally or nonverbally by the applicant in the introductory visit. Volunteers take brief notes after each session. These are useful for documentation of progress and for logistic reasons (e.g., someone having to fill in if regular volunteers are away). At the beginning and end of the program (week 2 and week 12), volunteers fill out a measure of the aphasic adult's participation in conversation [6]. Volunteers are trained to fill out this measure, which involves rating two areas—interaction (connection) and transaction (exchange of information, opinions, or feelings)—on a 9-point rating scale. The post-program rating is done twice, first without referring to the first rating and then with reference to this rating. There are pros and cons to both methods. Seeing a previous rating can have a biasing effect. On the other hand, giving a score just above a previous score says something specific in relation to change over time. We are exploring the use of functional communication measures, such as the American Speech-Language-Hearing Association Functional Assessment of Communication Skills for Adults [7].

At the end of the program, aphasic members, family members, and volunteers fill out program evaluation forms (Figure 11-3). Volunteers also have a "week 13," during which any ideas for improving the program are discussed. We have run six Introductory Programs so far and have continually upgraded the level of service by incorporating comments and suggestions from members, families, and volunteers.

CLINICAL TECHNIQUES

The Introductory Program has a psychosocial and psychoeducational agenda. The 12-week program (one morning session per week) is designed so that each session builds on the previous week, allowing participants to move through a process.

Four key elements are discussed:

- The group
- The volunteers
- The program format
- Program resources

The Group

At any given time, 20–25 aphasic members and their families participate in the program. The group is divided into smaller groups of four to five participants. Group selection was discussed earlier (see Entry Criteria).

The Volunteers

Volunteers are carefully recruited for this program from our existing volunteer pool. For the most part, those selected are among the most experienced and capable. Skill and experience are particularly important in this program because the group members are vulnerable and still in the early stages of dealing with the chronicity of aphasia.

A key feature of this program is that volunteers work in pairs and therefore must be comfortable with sharing the role of facilitator. Coleadership ensures continuity for the group, so that if one volunteer is away, the other can be present to ensure uninterrupted flow. We also try to have an extra "floater" volunteer to help out where there may be gaps.

In addition to the basic training described at the beginning of this chapter, volunteers receive specialized training in the following areas:

- Working in a coleadership relationship: Staff provide education and support to enable volunteers to share this leadership role.
- Training in the use of the rating scale administered in weeks 2 and 12.
- Understanding group stages: It is critical for volunteers to be aware of how groups evolve over time. This enables volunteers to watch for the evolution of trust and cohesiveness in their own group. Volunteers also

Name: _____   Term: 1   2   3   Year: _____

Please comment on your experience in the Introductory Program. Your comments will be helpful in planning future programs.

1. Was this a positive experience for you?   Y   N
   Please comment:

2. **Handover**
   a. Was the handover useful?   Y   N
   b. Are you happy with the format of the handover?   Y   N
   c. Are the reports useful?   Y   N
   d. Do you have any suggestions regarding the handover?

3. **Coleadership**
   a. Were you adequately prepared by staff to work in a   Y   N
      coleadership role?
   b. Is there anything else staff could have done to   Y   N
      prepare you or support you in this role?
   c. Did you have enough time to talk with your coleader?   Y   N
   d. Please tell us about the coleadership experience.

4. **Materials**
   a. Did you have sufficient materials (e.g., binders,   Y   N
      pictographic resources)?
   b. Were they helpful?   Y   N
   c. What other materials would be useful in a program
      like this?

5. **Group**
   Please comment on:
   a. Size

   b. Composition

   c. Peer session

      Was this useful for the group?   Y   N
      Do you have any suggestions for the peer session?

6. **Family Observation**
   Please comment briefly on how this went for the group and for you as a (co)leader. Please give us feedback on any other areas not covered above that will be important in planning other programs.

FIGURE 11-3.
Evaluation of Introductory Program: volunteer feedback.

Review Date: _____   Volunteer: _____

SLP: _____   Day(s) Attending: _____

To be completed by supervising SLP and volunteer:

Rate or Comment as Appropriate

Ability to facilitate a group (e.g., naturalness, use of humor)	0	1	2	3	4
Ability to co-facilitate	0	1	2	3	4
Effective listening skills	0	1	2	3	4
Flexibility (e.g., ability to adapt to group needs and changing circumstances)	0	1	2	3	4
Participation in volunteer meetings	0	1	2	3	4
Attendance and punctuality	0	1	2	3	4

General comments:

FIGURE 11-4.
Volunteer standards review. (SLP = speech-language pathologist.)

receive training in acting as "historians" for the group and maintaining awareness of chronology (e.g., "It is week 4, so there are eight more sessions to go").

- Understanding grief and loss: Volunteers are aware that many group participants are still in mourning. Staff provide volunteers with some education about the issues of loss.
- Starting a group session: Volunteers are given tools, specifically, warm-up activities, to help the group come together, focus, and get ready to work as a group. They are encouraged to use these activities at each session.
- Closure: This is an important aspect of group work at the Centre. Volunteers are taught to help the group reach closure and say good-bye. Members are encouraged to look back over the past 12 weeks and assess their progress.

The purpose of the volunteer meeting before each session begins is to help with preparation. The specific topic and resources or activities to facilitate the conversation of the day are covered. Volunteers are continually reminded about use of generic SCA techniques. The wrap-up meeting is a report back, giving volunteers the opportunity to discuss "magic moments" as well as discouraging ones; it also includes some preparation for the following week. Volunteers are always given time to talk with their coleaders before and after each program session. Staff are available for consultation and follow-up where required.

Based on our decision to invest in the intake process and the Introductory Program, there is a high staff-to-volunteer ratio. One speech-language pathologist is in charge and has a backup. A social worker participates in running the family group and also, where possible, in the preparatory and wrap-up volunteer sessions. Another speech-language pathologist participates as a consultant to the family group and gives feedback to the volunteers. This contrasts with the CAP program, where there is only one speech-language pathologist per 40–50 members, with access to speech-language pathology and social work backup only when resources allow.

Volunteers are carefully monitored as part of accountability and quality assurance. Because the volunteers are selected, we have not run into any serious difficulty. The Centre has recently developed a volunteer standards scale, which is now used routinely as part of the professional monitoring of this program (Figure 11-4).

The Program Format

Each session of the 12-week program is divided into two parts. First, members participate in a small "home" group for 1.25 hours. The small group enables members to explore specific material in a safe and comfortable environment. After this, all the groups get together for a half-hour in a large-group format. Family members finish their group at the same time and come out to join the large group. The

TABLE 11-1.
Example of Activities for the Introductory Program

Week Number	Activity	Comment
1–3	Telling stories	Members are encouraged to bring in photographs that help them "tell their story." This allows volunteers to get to know members well, so that even in the group setting there can be some programming for individual needs. Volunteers are encouraged to bring in photographs so that they, too, can share their stories.
	Signing the contract	Volunteers review a contract about the program with members which helps to clarify members' expectations.
	Talking about the definition of aphasia; beginning to think about setting goals	Volunteers help members revisit previous explanations about aphasia. This is done with the help of a resource booklet developed by the Centre. Note: Staff are always available to answer questions that come up in this section.
4–7	Communication	Volunteers help members engage in focused conversations about their communication. During these discussions, the members have a chance to become more aware of the strategies that they already use and to learn what others in the group find effective. In addition to these discussions, volunteers also work on communicative effectiveness.
8–10	Looking to the future	Members discuss goal setting, including both communication and general goals. At this point, staff introduce members to the idea of ongoing programming at the Centre. A unique feature of this module involves the use of peers. The peers are graduates of the Peer Support and Leadership Training Program offered at the Centre, which trains members who are experienced in living with aphasia. These experienced members share their insights and experiences with newer members.
11	Evaluation	The penultimate week of the program allows members to evaluate the program and their personal progress. This is an important week because it allows members to think back to the beginning of the program and helps them to consolidate what they have achieved.
12	Closure	Members have a chance to complete the program by saying good-bye to the home group through closure activities. They receive a certificate on this final day of the program. This explicit acknowledgment of the members as competent adult learners is invariably a highly emotional event that allows closure with the program as a whole.

purpose of the large group is to provide members with an opportunity to widen their social circle, thereby expanding the process of forming new *communities*.*

Groups use the outline shown in Table 11-1. The pace is always flexible. Groups of members with more severe aphasia take more time at certain stages.

The social worker is primarily responsible for running the family group. A speech-language pathologist is called in to work specifically on communication issues. During each Introductory Program, an evening session is held for extended family and friends of aphasic members so that

they too can learn more about aphasia, particularly about "masked competence" [1,2].

Program Resources

A distinguishing feature of our programming is that adults with severe aphasia are not excluded from conversations about complex topics. There may be differences in the pace and the depth at which the material is covered, but every participant has equal access to the subject matter, whatever the severity of aphasia. This is made possible by the following:

• The type of training given to the volunteers
• The use of specially designed resource material, which accompanies many discussions; most of the material is adapted from *Pictographic Communication Resources* [8]

We have learned from and been challenged by the Introductory Program in the following areas:

• Staff and volunteers have had to redefine the roles of helping and learning to balance opportunities for

---

*Here, the word *communities* refers to the many social networks to which we all belong (e.g., family, groups of friends or acquaintances with common bonds of history or special interests, work colleagues). The Centre has always been aware of the impact of social isolation that so often accompanies chronic aphasia, but we have thought either in terms of the loss of individual relationships or the loss of opportunity to participate in the community in its broad, abstract sense. We have now become more interested in small communities. We realize that, for many, the Introductory Program provides the first opportunity to re-establish a community. Our hope is that this is the first of many new communities inside and outside the Centre.

change and growth with support when change appears to be unlikely (e.g., for those with very severe chronic aphasia who might never be fluent speakers).

- We have seen the value of a closed-ended program where members have a pathway to follow, from a well defined starting point to a well defined end-point. This allows for a sense of achievement, accomplishment, and completion, and it contrasts with our old model, in which ongoing programs made it difficult to give a sense of movement and progress.

- We have benefited from the opportunity of working closely with social workers using a transdisciplinary model. This differs significantly from traditional parallel teamwork, in which certain issues become the domain of one discipline. With the transdisciplinary model, no single discipline has exclusive involvement in any particular area, although professional expertise comes into play in certain situations. This approach has positively affected the quality of our service.

DISCHARGE

The Centre's approach to discharge (namely, a policy of long-term support, with discharge decisions left largely to the member with aphasia and his or her family) is one of its unique features. Some years back, however, we arrived at a crisis point because of an increasing need for service with no increase in resources. It was then that we restructured our service, introducing the three-term system and a new method of intake that prepared applicants for enhanced participation at the Centre or in their own families and communities. With our current system, discharge can take place at three different points, the first being after the introductory visit, which we view as a conversation-based assessment as well as an intervention. This is the only point at which the discharge decision can be made by professional staff. Reasons relate to whether the applicant fits our entry criteria and will benefit from the program. Severity of aphasia, at either end of the continuum, is not one of our entry criteria. From this point on, aphasic members make their own decisions about discharge unless there is a change that affects the entry criteria. Thus, for example, we do not discharge someone because he or she has reached a plateau based on lack of documented progress on a standard measure of language or functional communication. We do consider discharge for a member who has developed a dementia that makes it difficult to function in the groups available at the Centre.

The second natural point of discharge for some members comes at the end of the 12-week Introductory Program. They are then eligible for the CAP, but some feel that they have gained what they came for or find that the program type is not for them. Not everyone enjoys being part of a group.

One advantage of our three-term system, particularly in the CAP, is that an aphasic member can choose to sign up or skip any particular term, just as any adult can do at a local community center. Members are given choices of activities each term and may not like the particular selection, may want to wait for space in a particular group (e.g., cooking), or may just want a break. This means that we are not left holding spaces, as used to happen with our old system. Members also do not have to worry about losing a space. When they are ready, they can participate once more, the only restriction being the availability of spaces in activities that interest them. These self-discharges are treated differently from a permanent decision to leave. Only if a member is away for a long period, especially if there have been any further complications, may he or she need to go through part of the intake process again.

Our system is working extremely well at present, and we have been able to handle the demand for service efficiently, without resorting to discharge in the traditional sense.

REIMBURSEMENT

When Pat Arato founded the Centre, it took 7 years to obtain funding from the Ontario Ministry of Health. During this time, the Centre survived solely on volunteer efforts, small donations of money and space, and typical grassroots funding efforts (e.g., bake sales). Currently, the Centre receives partial funding from the Ontario Ministry of Health. This partially covers rent and operating expenses, including the salaries of speech-language pathologists (three full-time employees) and administrative staff (executive director, volunteer coordinator, and office manager). Ministry funding does not fully cover these expenses, and certain positions (e.g., social work, program assistant, and some speech-language pathology positions) are not covered at all. The Centre relies on fundraising to cover these expenses and is currently seeking more secure funding.

The fact that we receive partial funding from the Ministry of Health precludes us from charging our aphasic members or families for anything related to the areas they fund (under the Canada Health Act). In other words, we are not allowed to charge for services such as our introductory visit and program, even though these involve expenses not covered by the Ministry. We therefore ask for tax-deductible donations from our members. The suggested amount at this time is Can $160 per term, which covers any services at any frequency.

CONCLUSION

Working at the Centre can be stressful for staff because our resources are often stretched to provide quality service to people with aphasia and their families. Additional stress relates to our inability to provide service to the thousands of aphasic people in Ontario who are living with aphasia and have no support. As staff, we need programs such as the one described in this chapter, because, in addition to providing a service, the programs also nourish and replenish our own sense of purpose in what we do. There are few dry eyes at the closing ceremony of the program, where we see people who hold themselves differently, show signs of genuine attachment to a new community of friends, and are beginning to see some kind of future for themselves.

Acknowledgments
Members with aphasia, families, volunteers, and staff at the Centre have all made invaluable contributions to the Introductory Program and, therefore, to this chapter. The format for the introductory visit that forms part of our intake process was developed by Lorraine Podolsky and Bea Bindman in consultation with staff. The authors would also like to acknowledge the contribution of Joe Rich to our understanding of group work.

REFERENCES

1. Kagan A, Winckel J, Shumway E. Supported conversation for aphasic adults. North York, Ontario: The Aphasia Centre–North York, 1995.
2. Kagan A. Supported conversation for adults with aphasia: methods and resources for training conversation partners. Aphasiology. (In press.)
3. Kagan A, Gailey GF. Functional Is Not Enough: Training Conversation Partners for Aphasic Adults. In AL Holland, MM Forbes (eds), Aphasia Treatment: World Perspectives. San Diego: Singular Publishing Group, 1993;199–225.
4. Jordan L, Kaiser W. Aphasia: A Social Approach. London: Chapman & Hall, 1996.
5. Parr S. The road more traveled: whose right of way? Aphasiology 1996;10:496–503.
6. Kagan A. Outcome measures from "supported conversation for adults with aphasia": preliminary psychometric evaluation and clinical applications. (In preparation.)
7. Frattali CM, et al. Functional Assessment of Communication Skills for Adults: ASHA FACS. Rockville, MD: American Speech-Language-Hearing Association, 1995.
8. Kagan A, Winckel J, Shumway E. Pictographic Communication Resources (manual). Toronto, Ontario: The Aphasia Centre–North York, 1996.

CHAPTER TWELVE

The Aphasia Self-Help Movement in Britain: A Challenge and an Opportunity

Ruth Coles and
Christine Eales

ACTION FOR DYSPHASIC ADULTS

Action for Dysphasic Adults (ADA) is a national charity formed 18 years ago by Diana Law, a businesswoman who was severely dysphasic* and wanted to provide more opportunities for language rehabilitation. In 1972, Ms. Law, with the help of a friend, wrote to the national press asking whether there were other people who were aphasic, unsupported, and interested in getting together to form speech clubs. She received more than 200 replies. Ms. Law worked from her London flat and traveled widely to talk about aphasia and to encourage the organization of speech clubs. At first, the emphasis was on forming local clubs with the assistance of speech and language therapists. It was some years before a London office was established with a professional adviser available to give information and advice.

At present, there are seven full- and part-time staff. The organization is still strongly supported by speech and language therapists, both on the staff and in a voluntary capacity as advisers and trustees, but in recent years people with dysphasia are taking a more central role in all aspects of ADA's work. ADA aims to educate both professional and lay people and to raise awareness of aphasia and its long-term effects. Through the membership of larger umbrella organizations, ADA lobbies for more resources and services. A telephone line for help and advice operates throughout the work week, and a range of literature, videotapes, and audiocassettes are available for people with aphasia and their families. There is a membership scheme with quarterly newsletters and an annual national conference. Legal and social advocacy is undertaken and assistance given to help people obtain services.

People with aphasia are represented on ADA's governing council; they also meet as a regional committee, which provides a vehicle for influencing policy decisions. The organization also holds strategic planning days, when people with dysphasia and family members work with council members and staff to draw up an action plan for a 3-year period.

The work of the charity has changed over the years, influenced both by the philosophy of the disability movement and by its own wish to move away from a paternalistic approach based on medical and philanthropic models of care. The social disability model offers new ideas for supporting people in living with aphasia [1]. As a voluntary organization with independent funding, ADA has provided a vehicle for exploring ways of putting ideas into practice.

In this chapter, we describe how these ideas have led ADA to support the development of self-help groups for people with aphasia. The organization has employed speech and language therapists in the role of regional development advisers to work with their colleagues in clinical practice to enable the setting up and supporting of self-help groups. Through the experience gained by the regional development advisers, we have evolved policies and a structure for their development and maintenance.

SELF-HELP AND THE DISABILITY MOVEMENT

The concept of self-help as a collection of individuals coming together to solve a common problem has a long history. It has served many purposes, from the improvement of housing and working conditions to the enfranchisement of women. It is in the second half of the twentieth century, however, that self-help has come of age in the fields of health and disability. The development of the Disability Movement, with its emphasis on self-determination, has had profound effects. Those who want to take control of their own lives and make decisions that affect them experience change, as do the professionals who are trained to assist them. To a smaller extent, so do the service providers, who are beginning to recognize the contribution self-help can make to recovery.

Some of the largest associations in Britain representing patient groups were initially formed by concerned relatives or parents of sick or disabled children. They were set up to raise public awareness of a condition and to ensure that appropriate services were provided. Many of these are now highly professional organizations run on business lines, with accountants, fundraisers, and political lobbyists. They may employ large numbers of volunteers; they contract out services and support major research projects into the prevention or treatment of particular medical conditions.

In Britain, the Stroke Association has for many years developed and funded volunteer-led speech groups and stroke clubs. These are based on a philanthropic model and are led largely by volunteers. They provide support to people with aphasia and their relatives through speech activities, friendship, and encouragement in a sheltered environment. Volunteers determine the structure of the therapy-type activities; people with dysphasia are the passive recipients. Although volunteers are largely untrained, their dysphasia support schemes receive statutory funding from the health authorities in the localities in which they operate.

It is perhaps because of this existing support that real self-help in Britain has got off to a slower start than in France, Germany, and Belgium. Germany and Belgium receive considerable statutory funding from local and national governments. The fast growth rate of self-help in other parts of Europe may reflect the lack of any aphasia therapy for most of the population. The European Commission set up a project known as *Helios*, through which it has provided money to enable voluntary organizations in the European member countries to meet to exchange information and learn from one another. As a result, the Association Internationale Aphasie has established itself as a focused resource through which members can share knowledge of all aspects of aphasia and of their activities in different countries.

---

*The terms *aphasia* and *dysphasia* are interchangeable in Britain.

THE SOCIAL MODEL OF DISABILITY
AND ITS APPLICATION TO APHASIA

The social model of disability defines disability as "the loss or limitation of opportunities that prevents people who have impairments from taking part in the normal life of the community on an equal level with others owing to physical and social barriers" [2]. It is proposed that these social barriers prevent people with aphasia from taking their normal place in the life of their families, friends, and the wider community.

Four types of barriers have been identified as disabling: environmental, structural, attitudinal, and informational. These barriers apply to aphasia as to any other disability.

- Environmental barriers are set up by the physical or language impairment.
- Structural barriers exist in the inability to obtain services and resources.
- Attitudinal difficulties are felt in the stigma that society attaches to people with a communication problem and the lack of awareness or understanding of aphasia.
- Informational barriers are present where the content or form of language material denies access or prevents full participation.

Aphasia Therapy and the Social Theory of Disability

Where the social theory of disability is accepted, a major shift in the focus of aphasia therapy has occurred. "Assessment and therapy focused on disability, when redefined in this way, must involve analysis of the restrictions encountered by aphasic people, and work on challenging, overcoming and changing *them*, rather than challenging and overcoming the impairment" [3].

Aphasia therapy has been provided by health and community services with the aim of treating the impairment and improving the level of language functioning. Some of the problems of proving the efficacy of functional therapy lie in the failure to understand the importance of social barriers surrounding impairment. Misunderstanding the significance of dismantling these barriers means that they are not measured as a factor in successful therapeutic intervention. Accepting the altered self after the onset of a disability and coming to terms with a new life with different power structures is ultimately the most important task for the affected individual. Speech and language therapists may well understand this, but it has not traditionally been recognized as a goal for therapy intervention. Financial constraints have dictated that clinical time is rarely invested in this way.

In this context, the development of self-help groups with complete autonomy for the aphasic members can be seen to offer an important opportunity for empowerment and self-determination. In describing the benefits to members of self-help groups, Wann [4] cites the ending of isolation, sharing personal experiences of pain and anger, and finding practical solutions to problems. The atmosphere of openness allows taboo subjects to be aired in trust and confidence.

Matzat [5] defines self-help groups as follows:

In self-help groups, all members are affected and come into direct contact with one another. Their activities are on a local basis and oriented directly to the state of needs of their members. They are small groups, facilitating face-to-face contact and discussion. Contacts are spontaneous, little organised, and lively. The structure of these groups is unstable, and often they are short lived.

SPEECH AND LANGUAGE THERAPISTS
AND SELF-HELP GROUPS

For clinicians, aphasia self-help groups are an additional resource offering further opportunities to extend the network of long-term support outside the clinical setting: "Therapists see that the groups provide a natural opportunity for using and developing communication gains made in therapy. These groups also offer a means of exploring and developing a range of skills and roles not promoted in the "culture" of therapy" [6]. Group members contribute their personal experiences and are uniquely able to help each other come to terms with living with aphasia. Emotional burdens can be shared and people can be enabled and empowered to establish a new identity, recognizing their disability but maintaining their former sense of self. For the therapist, helping a client to join a peer group implies a healthy letting go. Wann [4] recognizes this particular benefit: "Reaching out to those with a shared experience breaks away from being a victim encouraged to refer to experts for help." Robinson [7] stated, "Members of autonomous self-help groups are empowered not only because they learn by doing but also because they are changed by doing."

Clinicians live in the real world of limited resources. They know that the time available to work with the language impairment and help the client come to terms with it is "unlikely to span the period during which the aphasic person ceases to understand the condition as an illness and starts to take it on as a disability" [8]. In assisting the development of self-help groups for people with aphasia, a clinician ensures a forum for working through issues that will arise when the client is no longer in contact with speech-language therapy services.

HOW SELF-HELP GROUPS DIFFER
FROM THERAPY GROUPS

The practicing clinician concerned with the transfer of therapeutic strategies into everyday language activities may offer the aphasic client a period in a language-based therapy group. Such a group provides opportunities for normal automatic social language, rituals of greeting, and acknowledging and lessens the artificiality of language-based therapy tasks. In a hospital or clinic group, however, the speech therapist normally takes the lead. In spite of the environment of support and mutual encouragement, the power lies not with the group members but with the clinician who controls and leads the group. Such groups may provide a valuable therapeutic tool, but they are fulfilling a different function from the autonomy that develops in a self-help group.

A CHANGE IN THE BALANCE OF POWER

Jordan and Kaiser examined aphasia from three perspectives: people with dysphasia, policies, and power [9]. They distinguish between *power to* and *power over*: "*Power to* may mean the ability to achieve a desired end or to influence others. *Power over* another person or group implies the ability to impose your will even against the wishes or the interests of the others." The sense of powerlessness and dependency that develops in someone with aphasia after a stroke requires the clinician's "power to." This may mean assisting the aphasic client to take the next step toward autonomy as therapy draws to an end.

Rootes and Aanes [10] set out seven points to define a self-help group:

- A self-help group is supportive and educational.
- Leadership comes from within the group.
- The group addresses a single major life-disrupting event.
- Group members participate voluntarily.
- The group has no monetary interest or profit orientation.
- The primary purpose of group membership is individual personal growth.
- Membership is anonymous and confidential.

THE FIRST APHASIA SELF-HELP GROUP

The first self-help group established by a clinician for people with aphasia was set up in Harrow, North London, by Mandyle May, a speech and language therapist who saw self-help as flowing naturally from speech-language therapy. She recognized that the group would offer a place for people to practice learned skills in an accepting environment and provide opportunities for the recovery of self-confidence and empowerment through people assuming specific tasks within the group. As a clinician working with a full caseload, she also recognized the benefit to the therapist: "Through . . . empowering people to take responsibility for their own support structures, the group has reduced the amount of therapy resources needed" [11].

The Harrow group took some months to coalesce, slowly developing an assertiveness that was to find its expression in collective action. Group members were worried about crossing a busy road to reach their meeting place and visited members of their local council to ask for a pedestrian crossing. They felt greatly empowered when, as result of their visit, the council acted to make the road safer. The confidence that grew from this success led to other activities, such as the printing and sale of a Christmas card designed by a member and the holding of an art exhibition in the local hospital. The group has successfully dismantled some

of the social barriers described earlier and has grown in personal and collective confidence in the process.

When this group became affiliated with the ADA, the value of self-help became apparent. It was decided that ADA should make the encouragement of self-help a priority and appoint speech and language therapists as regional development advisers to assist in establishing self-help groups.

For these clinicians, supporting the setting up and maintenance of self-help groups has meant a fundamental change of approach and has proved a challenging and invigorating experience. Although there is a growing literature on self-help theory, experiential learning rather than formal training has been the most effective support in the early stages [12].

INVOLVEMENT IN SELF-HELP: IMPLICATIONS FOR THE THERAPIST

Involvement in the life issues of an aphasic person has not traditionally been seen as the responsibility of the speech and language therapist, whose work has largely been concerned with the language deficit. The therapist who wishes to work in this way may have to challenge the traditional pattern of service provision. Funding may be difficult until the benefits are clearly established. In Britain, the employment of a voluntary organization has provided one opportunity for development. In another instance, the study of the benefit of self-help has been presented as a project that has successfully attracted research funding.

ISSUES FOR THE THERAPIST IN ESTABLISHING A GROUP

To start a self-help group, it is necessary to have two or three interested people with aphasia. One of them must have sufficient language skills to take the lead. They are likely to need assistance with practical matters, such as helping to find a suitable space, obtaining transport, and publicizing themselves to attract other members. At first, members may have difficulty deciding on such simple issues as where and when to meet. The therapist must have time and patience to facilitate discussion and allow the gradual building of confidence. The therapist needs to commit time, possibly for up to a year, to help the group understand the nature of self-help, explore what they hope to achieve, and develop aims for the group.

As a professional, the speech and language therapist has held the power in the therapeutic relationship through knowledge and acquired skills. Facilitation of a self-help group demands the development of new skills. The clinician-client relationship must give way to an equal partnership in which the therapist and the person with aphasia can learn from each other. The therapist helps the group to proceed at its own pace and allows it to take risks and to make mistakes. As the group grows in confidence and assertiveness, members may decide that they do not wish to have a professional at their meetings. This rejection may be painful, but it marks progress for the group and should be celebrated by the therapist. It may also be difficult when the result of enabling people with aphasia is to empower them to be highly critical of the service they have received.

ISSUES FOR MEMBERS OF A GROUP

Members have to accept that they have ownership of the group and not depend on the therapist to make decisions for them. This involves understanding the therapist's new role as facilitator and enabler. Members require time to learn to recognize the therapist as a resource on which the group can draw. They must learn how to communicate with one another and understand each other's communication systems. They need to establish turn taking and may develop rules for the conduct of meetings. Groups develop very different identities, depending on the personalities of the members.

GOALS

Different ADA groups identify different aims and achieve different goals. Members of one group regularly speak at conferences and disability forums, thereby raising the awareness of aphasia and educating professionals. Another group has sent letters to health care planners, highlighting the need for an improvement in therapy provision. One group has targeted local stores, explaining language impairment to shop staff and awarding a sticker to be displayed in the shop window of enlightened participants. All of these are examples of the disabling barriers that the groups come to identify for themselves as they grow in confidence.

PRACTICAL GUIDELINES

Two sets of booklets [13] have been developed, providing separate guidance for people with dysphasia and for speech and language therapists interested in starting groups. One covers practical matters, such as forming a group, finding accommodation, and opening a bank account. Another deals with sharing responsibilities, developing aims, planning activities, and overcoming some of the problems that arise in groups. The Nottingham self-help team, which is the leading self-help center in the United Kingdom, has been an excellent source of research knowledge and provided a wealth of experience. Their publications and start-up packs are recommended to our groups. An invaluable resource for the regional development advisers is *How to Work with Self-Help Groups—Guidelines for Professionals* [14].

SELF-HELP WORKSHOPS

ADA has held two workshops in London to enable speech and language therapists and people with aphasia to form a working partnership to explore the philosophy of self-help and its practical implications in developing a group.

The stages in the life cycle of a group, as described in a model by Tuckman [15], were explored, and therapists and members of existing groups related their experiences. It proved reassuring for these groups to see that the tribulations they may have experienced conform to Tuckman's four stages (forming, storming, norming, and performing) and that other kinds of self-help groups also experience them.

One group who approached ADA never developed from the initial forming stage. People in a short-term residential rehabilitation center would form a group, begin to get to know one another and to talk about their aphasia, and then return home and cease contact. The group served only as short-term support, with the therapist remaining as group leader; the group never became independent.

One ADA group leader described many stormy patches. "Storming" occurred early on, when it was decided that relatives should no longer attend meetings, and later, when conflicts of interest arose and half the members left to join a therapist-led group in the same locality. The group later reached the performing stage: functioning well, looking to support people with aphasia, and creating awareness of the condition in their local community.

EXPERIENCES OF GROUP MEMBERS

Setting up a self-help group is hard enough when you are able-bodied, but when you have a disability which means you have a language disorder, it's a challenge. (Cressida Laywood, Nottingham group, personal communication, 1997)

My first meeting with the self-help group . . . was . . . I didn't want to be part of it. I was looking for people who were . . . my colleague types, who were able to communicate and outward going. But it's changed my life, meeting people at the self-help group, because they were bright, many of them very bright, successful people before their strokes, and they're re-adapting again as I am to a totally new life, and being very positive . . . the self-help group helped me a lot. (Margot Larkin, Central London Group [16])

Alan Hewitt and Cressida Laywood have aphasia. They are founding members and leaders of groups in Gateshead and Nottingham and have given each other considerable support. The following provides their own insights about sclf-help groups:

Because we founded the groups with a lot of support from professionals and families, we had a great influence on the policies and practices of our two groups. Although there are different ways of setting up a self-help group, we both feel it needs a person with aphasia who is *motivated* enough to want to do it. Apart from all the existential factors which will affect the success of the group, it needs to be the right person, so don't rush it. . . . Self-help groups can provide support to people who are very isolated because of their disability—however, it is important to realise that people with aphasia need to think whether they have the emotional stamina to [get] the challenge. (A. Hewitt and C. Laywood, personal communication, 1997)

Hewitt and Laywood feel that researching other groups was very important for the success of their two groups:

As the groups develop, they can be fine-tuned. A dynamic group is always changing; however, there needs to be a structure to the group and the meetings, a structure to the relationship between the group and the speech and language therapist, and a structure to the relationship between the group and ADA. The regional development advisers are the go-betweens, forging new relationships between people with aphasia and the [local] speech and language therapists.

Hewitt and Laywood suggest that groups adopt policies on the following issues:

- Whether to have an *open* policy (people with aphasia and their caregivers) or a *closed* policy (people with aphasia only)
- How many people to allow in the group
- Ratio of men to women
- Age of members (e.g., Nottingham only accepts those who are younger than 65 years old)

Hewitt and Laywood state:

In Nottingham there is a closed policy, in Gateshead there is an open policy. In Gateshead, although the number of people with dysphasia is about the same (10–12), the chairing of the meeting has to be tighter, to stop [caregivers] talking in place of people with aphasia. The severity of the aphasia is not a bar, but there needs to be a person in the group who has just enough language skills to organise the group. In both cases, we try to be very clear about our aims and objectives. They are to get people with dysphasia communicating among themselves first of all, then to get the group out into the community, and to provide all the support they need to do it.

REGIONAL DEVELOPMENT ADVISERS

The qualified therapists who work for ADA as regional development advisers support a network of self-help groups, visiting them when requested, and providing help in times of transition or crisis. They facilitate the early discussions and make it possible for all the members to express their views. They assist groups in forming a committee and opening a bank account. When groups affiliate to the national body, they are given a start-up grant to help with the early expenses of running a group. The regional development advisers provide ADA literature and posters that the group can use for recruitment or for local awareness-raising events. They may offer assistance in making links with local radio or help with press releases. Groups may be helped to develop aphasia-friendly materials for their meetings, such as building photographic records of their activities. The work of Kagan and Gailey [17] at the Pat Arato Aphasia Centre in North York, Ontario, Canada, has influenced the development of aphasia-friendly presentations and newsletters.

LIAISON WITH SPEECH AND LANGUAGE THERAPISTS

For the practicing clinician, establishing a good working relationship with the groups is important, as Hewitt and Laywood recognize (personal communication, 1997):

The self-help group puts a new slant on the relationship between the clinician and the people with aphasia. It carries the work of the speech and language therapist more deeply into the community, and means that there are people with aphasia for the first time in the disability/voluntary sector movement.

The local speech and language therapist is a valuable link for the group and acts as the agency for referring new members. Some therapists enjoy keeping in touch with a group and may accept an invitation to become honorary committee members. Therapists who support the establishment of self-help groups may advise each other using ADA as a network. Some groups ask the local therapist to screen potential members; others accept direct contact from new members.

NETWORKING OPPORTUNITIES FOR SELF-HELP GROUPS

ADA groups are able to share information about their experiences with one another by sending representatives to regional committee meetings. These meetings also offer an opportunity to discuss national issues and to influence the policy of the national organization. The assertiveness of established groups and the campaigning and awareness projects in which they are involved show up the hesitancy and anxieties of newer groups. Chairing the meetings is demanding, and the aphasic chairperson works with the staff in preparing the agenda. Some members need facilitators to assist them with issues they wish to raise. Members have adopted rules of conduct, such as not interrupting a speaker. Minutes of the meetings are produced in large type, with lots of space and simple sentence construction. Information from the groups is included in a newsletter twice a year. Considerable use is made of symbols and pictures to overcome the information barrier and to make these documents as accessible as possible (Figure 12-1).

COMMITTEE MEMBERS' WORKING PARTY

One self-help initiative has been the creation of a working party to look at the Disability Discrimination Act of 1995 and study how it will affect people with aphasia (Figure 12-2). The group has accepted the assistance of a facilitator and scribe. In practice, this help has proved essential in clarifying issues among members and preventing misinterpretation. Abstract discussion is both difficult and tiring for people with aphasia, but the group has already covered many facets of the law and is on target to complete its task. The national organization has actively encouraged this initiative and provided a grant to enable the work to be done.

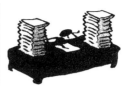

Action for Dysphasic Adults
Self Help Groups
newsletter no.2

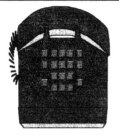

0171-261-9572

Welcome to the second ADA self -help group newsletter.

The Regional Development Advisers (**Chris** and **Gill)** have looked at all the criticism of the last newsletter and hope we have improved.

This time we feature two groups one from the North **Preston** and one from the South **HASH**.This will become a regular feature so please be ready for your turn.

Please read, enjoy and share with others

Raising **Awareness**

• **Worthing** have had discussions with Virgin Airlines on air travel and the needs of people with dysphasia.They are soon to meet with their customer relations manager.

• Most groups take part in local charity and health promotion events.

• Following a request from **Brighton** the Regional Committee have asked ADA to look at producing banners, sashes,T-shirts,lapel badges to help the groups promote awareness of dysphasia.

• **Brighton** were involved in a"health care fun day"

• **Nottingham** group have been involved in:
CVS Charity Fair.
Gelding CVS ADA and the Stroke Association event and,Nottingham City Council Look Lively event.

• **Phaser (Cornwall)** manned a stall at Cornwall's 4th July charity event

• **Cambridge** had stalls at Fulbourn Hospital May Fayre and Charity Bazaar in the Guildhall.

FIGURE 12-1.
Action for Dysphasic Adults Self-Help Groups newsletter.

PROBLEMS

Both theory and practice of self-help in aphasia is still evolving. Much remains to be learned, given that the very medium in which groups normally communicate with one another is the site of the disability. The social skills of welcoming a member and helping the individual to settle in may not be available to the group. Misunderstandings arise, and it is easy for people to hurt one another unintentionally. One member said, "I can't wrap it up any more, I can only tell it straight." Arrangements for meetings and outings can be casualties of imprecise language. People bring different expectations to groups, and some may go away disappointed. Some people are unwilling or unable to recognize the need for facilitation. Others find great difficulty in accepting another person's handicap. Groups of people with aphasia face the same problems as other groups, such as an insensitive or domineering leader. We are still evolving ways of helping members to overcome these difficulties. A series of group skills workshops is in preparation, wherein members can learn strategies to help their groups function better.

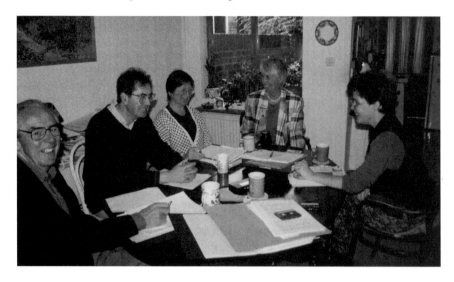

FIGURE 12-2.
Disability Discrimination Act working party.

CONCLUSION

Our experiences are based on the development of 15 self-help groups in a 3-year period. Despite the difficulties, it is clear that self-help provides many people with a valuable vehicle to make the necessary changes to adapt to the disability of aphasia. For speech and language therapists who embrace self-help and assist people to dismantle the barriers caused by aphasia, the work is challenging, instructive, and rewarding. Listening to what people with aphasia themselves require may influence service planning and inform new initiatives in service delivery.

For a voluntary organization, encouragement of self-help is a logical development. We seek an effective channel for communicatively impaired people to inform and direct our activities. The goal for those with aphasia, and for the professionals and voluntary organizations assisting them, is to dismantle the barriers that frustrate and disable people. Self-help can provide an effective model for empowering people to do this for themselves as well as a valuable means of increasing knowledge and understanding for those of us involved in its development. Overcoming the difficulties that occur in the process is proving to be a challenge well worth meeting.

Acknowledgments
We are grateful to Alan Hewitt and Cressida Laywood, who have contributed their experiences, and to Sally Byng, Susie Parr, and Carole Pound of The City University, London, who are forging a new chapter in understanding and meeting the needs of people with aphasia.

REFERENCES

1. Pound C. New approaches to long term aphasia therapy and support. Bulletin of the Royal College of Speech and Language Therapists 1996;532:12–13.
2. Finklestein V, French S. Towards a Psychology of Disability. In J Swain, V Finklestein, S French, M Oliver (eds), Disabling Barriers—Enabling Environments. London: OU Publications and Sage, 1993;9–61.
3. Parr S. Everyday literacy in aphasia: radical approaches to functional assessment and therapy. Aphasiology 1996;5:469–479.
4. Wann M. Building Social Capital: Self Help in the Twenty-First Century Welfare State. London: Institute for Public Policy Research, 1995;51.
5. Matzat J. Self-help groups as basic care in psychotherapy and social work. Groupwork 1989–1990;2:248–256.
6. Pound C. Accessing aphasia: developing disability level therapies. Presented to the British Aphasiology Society, Manchester, England, September 1997.
7. Robinson D. Self-help groups in primary health care. World Health Forum 1981;2:183–191.
8. Parr S. The road more travelled, whose right of way? Aphasiology 1996;10:496–503.
9. Jordan L, Kaiser W. Aphasia—A Social Approach. London: Chapman, 1996.
10. Rootes LE, Aanes DL. A conceptual framework for understanding self-help groups. Hospital and Community Psychiatry 1992;43:379–381.
11. Le May M. Group Dynamics. Therapy Weekly December 2, 1993.
12. Katz AH, Hedrick HL (eds). Self-Help Concepts and Applications. San Diego: San Diego Press, 1992;58.
13. Wisdom C. Self-Help Guidelines for Professionals. London: ADA Publications, 1996.
14. Nottingham Self-Help Team Publications. Nottingham, England: Nottingham Self-Help, 1995.
15. Tuckman BW. Developmental sequences in small groups. Psychol Bull 1965;63:384–399.
16. Personal Insights Audiocassette. London: ADA Publications, 1995.
17. Kagan A, Gailey GF. Functional Is Not Enough: Training Conversation Partners for Aphasic Adults. In AL Holland, MM Forbes (eds), Aphasia Treatment—World Perspectives. San Diego, CA: Singular Publishing Group, 1993;199–225.

CHAPTER THIRTEEN

The Power of Aphasia Groups

Audrey L. Holland
and Roger Ross

There was a time in the not-distant past when I (ALH) believed that group treatment was a useful adjunct to individual treatment for chronically aphasic adults. I have changed my mind. I now believe that individual treatment is a useful adjunct to group treatment for such patients. The reasons for my change of perspective are many, and I have been influenced by the points of view of many other contributors to this book, including Aura Kagan, Marjorie Graham, Robert Marshall, and Roberta Elman. The major influences on my thinking in this regard, however, have been aphasic individuals themselves and the features of the rehabilitation process that have been most influential in their recovery. One of the most influential of these individuals is the coauthor of this chapter, whose previous writings on group treatment are featured here. In this chapter, I take the primary responsibility for constructing these sentences, but Roger Ross has done most of the thinking behind them.

> I have a sense that, after my stroke, I did not get better until I met other people with the same problem. My colleagues and I believe that joining a group is the most important thing that a stroke survivor can do for himself or herself. [1]

This belief is shared by most of the people who come to aphasia groups at the University of Arizona. Why? What is the unique healing ingredient in groups? We wish to explore their power in this chapter. We harbor the belief that, with understanding, we might be able to find ways to translate this power to individual treatment as well.

Despite how much clinicians may have read about aphasia, language, and communication or interacted with aphasic talkers in clinical encounters, an unassailable fact is that very few clinicians have actually been there themselves. The essence of aphasia is its uniqueness. Few other problems that humans encounter are quite so exotic, so pervasive, so unexpected, so baffling in their variability. Many aspects of aphasic language have analogues in normal language functioning, such as occasional difficulties in retrieving words or in understanding what a particularly opaque speaker may be attempting to communicate. These problems are transient, though, and for the most part not to be taken very seriously. These analogues may help a clinician to understand the problems of aphasia a bit better, but they offer little in the way of explanations that help the aphasic speaker.

One of the most important group powers is that group members are far more likely to be empathetic with each other than are either families or clinicians. Group members' own experiences have prepared them to understand very well the frustrations, anger, depression, and vexation that result from aphasia. Even when group members have different types of aphasia, have different levels of severity, or have different amounts of experience at being aphasic, we can assume that they share its almost universal ill effects. Clinicians must try to understand, and many excellent clinicians do come close, but the fact that their clinicians have not lived these problems is obvious to most individuals with aphasia. The highest degree of empathy comes from those who have shared the experience.

Empathy alone does not explain the power of the aphasia group, however. The group makes other unique contributions to the recovery process, as well as to the longer-term process of living with residual aphasia. The support that group members can provide for each other has many facets. One particularly notable advantage of the group experience is that aphasic individuals frequently can share personal solutions to their problems that have the gold-plated guarantee of having worked. For example, while observing one of Roger's self-run aphasia groups, I watched people with widely different types and degrees of aphasia share with each other (via speech, gesture, writing, and inflectional and prosodic changes) a number of workable solutions to a common problem: difficulty in sleeping through the night. In the first place, I had no idea that sleeping problems were common in aphasia, yet all 12 people in this group were bothered by them. I also suspect that had I thought to bring up sleeping problems with an aphasia group before witnessing this very helpful interchange, I would have invited in an "expert" to talk to them about the problem.

Another example comes from a group in our University of Arizona clinic in which Roger Ross participates. The youngest member of this group, Herb, was going for a job interview, and the other group members decided to help him practice for it. (In fact, every member of this group except Herb had had experience hiring other people.) My role was to watch and comment. I watched the interviews and the subsequent criticisms with growing horror, for Herb's questioners were very hard on him, and the feedback was particularly forceful and direct. Herb did not seem disturbed by it but appeared to be taking it very well. I intervened nonetheless. And the group told me quite pointedly that if Herb expected to get the job, he was going to have to be far more sure of himself than he was acting. Particularly because he had a language problem, they argued, he had to demonstrate his ability to handle this job in a strong and forthright manner. Herb clearly understood the support that underlay the group's remarks, and I did not. Does it surprise the reader to find out that Herb got the job?

In terms of communication, group members sometimes provide "encouragement" that no clinician would regard as beneficial. For example, Jon, a member of a group in our clinic, is almost totally nonverbal and relies on a number of other strategies, particularly drawing, for communication. Another member of his group, Bill, frequently urges him to "come on now, say it." Far from being frustrated by Bill's urging, Jon appears to take it as an article of Bob's faith in him, and they share a strong bond of friendship that seems in some way to be built on it.

I believe this ability to challenge, to push each other to try new things, and to encourage risk taking is uniquely useful between aphasic people. I sometimes find myself catching my breath as I watch the process, knowing that I would never have the gumption to try some of the things with aphasic individuals that Roger does. He is, in his words, "very, very tough." For example, he told me that he had advised an aphasic woman in his group in Scottsdale that she simply had to do some of the physical activities that have become frightening since her stroke. He believes it is critical for her to confront the wariness, accept its challenge, and require herself to overcome it. He believes this is part of the recovery process. Is *gumption* the right term? Both Roger and I are probably essentially correct in the way we behave. I do not have the right to make the demands that Roger and his fellow aphasic group members make of each other. I have never been there. I am an outsider to this part of the therapeutic power of aphasia groups.

Then there is the group experience itself. Roger Ross and I have shared some incidents in which individuals with right hemisphere impairments came to an aphasia group, with somewhat distressing results. The aphasic group members found their talking time to be severely compromised, along with their sense of control over the situation itself. They had been usurped, or at least disenfranchised. This is in stark contrast to what both of us believe to be a particularly satisfying feature of aphasia groups. Its members have a strong sense of empowerment. Roger has written elsewhere that new members of a group tell their stories of stroke and rehabilitation and how every story tells the rest of the group something new. Effective members of the group (not the nonaphasic facilitators) make certain that all participate in the talking, and everyone listens respectfully and attentively to others' contributions. There is an energy to aphasia groups that is driven by members, not by the facilitator.

One term, when we were a little short of student trainees, Pelagie Beeson and I decided that our high-functioning group (their self-designation) actually did not need a student clinician. We had spent the preceding term shushing the student anyway. When we made this announcement, not a second elapsed before one of the members said, "I thought it was our job to educate your students." The group had their student for the next session. In this particular group, sometimes the sense of aphasic empowerment can be overwhelming to even the most resilient of nonaphasic group facilitators. Those of us who used to think we had some say in the group's activities have long ago accepted our roles as occasional advisors and frequent secretaries. We consider ourselves lucky to be invited to attend. Because of their shared experiences, their empathy, and their knowledge of what aphasia is all about, their social isolation melts away for at least an hour, and the serious business of shared concerns can be dealt with.

Roger and I both believe that there is no end to the need for such aphasia groups. There is a sort of lifetime perspective to the group's existence, and the need for it is much like the need for continuing the other things one does to maintain a healthy and vigorous life. This was beautifully illustrated in Roger's group, which had just accepted a man named Arthur who was relatively newly aphasic. Arthur was voicing his great frustration at how slowly he was progressing. In particular, he complained about how difficult it was to be stuck at reading at a slow pace, far from his prestroke reading level. How long, he asked, would he have to be coming to aphasia group? At least three members of this group had similar problems, and through long, hard, and constant self-disciplined practice had regained the ability to read again for pleasure. These three members looked at each other, and a long pause followed. Cheryl, typically the most diplomatic member, swallowed hard, looked to her fellow group members for support, and said, "Get used to this group, Arthur. You're here for life." At least 6 months have elapsed since then. Arthur is still coming, his reading is improving, and he is traveling and beginning to enjoy life again. We think that this is the power of aphasia groups.

Acknowledgment

This work was supported in part by National Multipurpose Research and Training Center Grant DC01409 from the National Institute on Deafness and Other Communication Disorders.

REFERENCES

1. Ross R. Aphasia groups: a view from the inside. Advance Magazine, May 3, 1966:18.

SECTION III

Right Hemisphere Damage

CHAPTER FOURTEEN

Group Treatment for Patients with Right Hemisphere Damage

Leora R. Cherney
and Anita S. Halper

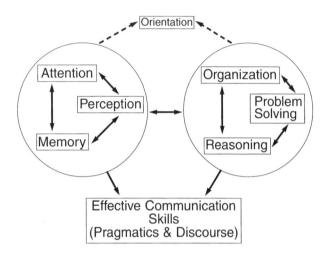

FIGURE 14-1.
Schematic representation of interrelationships among cognitive processes.

PHILOSOPHY OF PROGRAM

Damage to the right hemisphere results in a cluster of cognitive deficits that reduces the patient's effective and efficient communication skills. Such cognitively based disorders of communication have been referred to as *cognitive-communicative impairments* [1]. A conceptual framework for the clinical management of cognitive-communicative impairments associated with right hemisphere damage has grown out of our clinical experience of more than 20 years with this population. Figure 14-1 is a schematic representation of the interrelationships of various cognitive processes that may be affected by right hemisphere damage [2]. It is not intended to be a theoretical model of brain organization and function, but is meant as a clinical guide for selecting appropriate evaluation and treatment materials.

The premise of the framework is that the processes of attention, perception, memory, organization, reasoning, and problem solving underlie the performance of any functional behavior, including communication. When communication breaks down in a specific task, the underlying reason must be analyzed. Depending on the results of the analysis, the clinician may choose to work on the presumed underlying impaired cognitive processes (process-specific approach), the impaired cognitive-communicative behaviors that result from these deficits (functional approach), or both.

The process-specific and functional approaches can be effectively delivered via group treatment. In addition, the teaching of strategies to compensate for the underlying impairment or to improve functional performance are an integral part of both approaches and can be incorporated into group treatment for the patient with right hemisphere damage. Regardless of the treatment approach, generalization is an essential component, and groups provide a vehicle for facilitating this process.

Group treatment is a cost-effective means of providing quality care, particularly considering the impact of health care and the limited financial resources that might be available to the patient. For example, many insurance companies reimburse on a per diem basis regardless of the frequency and mode of treatment. Therefore, from the provider standpoint, the cost of delivering treatment in groups is less because more patients can be seen at one time.

Group treatment is an appropriate method of delivering speech-language pathology services to patients with right hemisphere damage at all levels of care (inpatient, outpatient, day rehabilitation, long-term care). Regardless of differences in patient and family goals, discharge placement, and severity of cognitive-communicative impairment, common outcome goals at each level of care permit the development of groups specific to that level. At the Rehabilitation Institute of Chicago (RIC) System of Care, a number of groups have evolved for patients with right hemisphere damage.

Table 14-1 lists the types of groups that are used at each level of care at the RIC. Although long-term care is not currently part of the RIC System of Care, group treatment of patients with right hemisphere problems is an appropriate mode of treatment delivery in that setting and has been included in Table 14-1.

The following section provides an overview of each group listed in Table 14-1, including admission criteria, frequency of group sessions, and recommended size. We believe that the minimum size of any group should be three scheduled patients. Because cancellations are frequent, groups that are formed with fewer than three patients may sometimes have only one or two participants. This affects group dynamics as well as economics.

For each group discussed, a table is provided as a quick reference for clinicians to use in the group treatment of patients with cognitive-communicative deficits after right hemisphere damage. The tables provide an overall goal, a list of some of the variables that can be manipulated or measured, and functional group treatment activities for each skill area. The goals provide a skeleton structure in which components such as objective measures, levels of activity, and specific environments can be added. These goals can be modified to serve as either long-term or short-term goals. The tables are based on treatment ideas developed from our clinical experience and on what we believe is optimal for this patient population. They are intended as a guide rather than an exhaustive list of treatment options for this population.

ORIENTATION GROUP

The orientation group focuses on cognitive processes that directly affect orientation, namely, attention, memory, and perception. The following skills are stressed in this group:

- Sustained and selective attention
- Attention to the left hemispace
- Remembering personal biographical information

TABLE 14-1.
Types of Groups at Each Level of Care

	Subacute Rehabilitation	Acute Rehabilitation	Outpatient Rehabilitation	Day Rehabilitation	Long-Term Care
Orientation group	X	X			X
High-level cognitive group		X	X	X	
Pragmatics group	X	X	X	X	X
Life skills group			X	X	

- Perception of environmental cues
- Using simple orientation compensatory strategies, such as a watch, daily schedule, and calendar

All of these skills facilitate orientation to time, place, and person.

Patients must meet one of two criteria for admission to this group: (1) a rating of severe (raw score of 13 or less out of a possible 24) on the Behavioral Observation Profile of the RIC Evaluation of Communication Problems in Right Hemisphere Dysfunction–Revised (RICE-R) (Figure 14-2) or (2) an overall rating of moderately severe or severe on the RIC Rating for Cognitive-Communicative Deficits in Right Hemisphere Dysfunction (Table 14-2).

It is preferable that this group be held daily (including weekends, if available) for an hour either at the beginning or end of the day. This allows a discussion of the day's activities, either to help members get ready for the day or provide closure to the day. Some facilities may choose to conduct an orientation group at both times of the day, for a half-hour each. The group should consist of a minimum of three and a maximum of six patients with one speech-language pathologist. The distractibility and impulsivity of group participants are factors to consider in determining optimum size.

Table 14-3 illustrates a variety of activities appropriate for orientation group. Certain activities are performed routinely, including perception of environmental cues to orient the patient to time and place and sharing personal biographical information. As the patients improve, task variables to increase the level of difficulty are manipulated.

To illustrate how variables are manipulated on an ongoing basis according to the individual patient's level of functioning, consider the goal of improving sustained and selective attention. For this goal, it is important to choose activities that the patient can perform, so that the focus is on improving attention rather than accuracy of performance. For the activity of reading the patient's hospital menu, the task is to select meals for the next day and discuss their selection with the other patients. To manipulate the variable of length, one patient may be given the whole day's menu whereas another is given the items of just one meal. To manipulate the input mode, one patient can read the menu to the other patients; some patients have the written menu in front of them and others receive only the auditory information. Depending on the patients' performance, distracters can be introduced. These distracters

may include opening the door to the treatment room, taking a telephone call, or adding pictures to the wall or items on the tabletop. The activity could take place in a quiet treatment room or in a hospital dining room. Visual and auditory cues to redirect the patient back to the task may be provided. The clinician can measure the time each patient attends to the menu-reading task and the number of cues needed for redirection. Similarly, during discussion of each patient's menu selection, the same variables can be measured.

Increasing awareness of memory problems is an essential part of the group's focus of using simple compensatory strategies to retain orientation information. At times, the clinician may have to set up situations that highlight the patient's memory problem. For example, the patient can be asked to remember a piece of information or complete a task for a period during which it is known that he or she will forget. Soliciting feedback from group participants may help reinforce the patient's awareness of this problem.

HIGH-LEVEL GROUP

The high-level cognitive group focuses on the processes of organization, reasoning, problem solving, and memory. Skills stressed in this group are these:

- Effective use of compensatory memory strategies in a more natural setting
- Organization, sequencing, and prioritization of information pertinent to real-life situations
- Analysis and identification of appropriate solutions to functional problems

These skills permit the patient to achieve greater independence at home, in the community, and at work, if appropriate.

Patients must meet one of two criteria for admission to this group: (1) a rating of mild (raw score of 19 or more out of a possible 24) on the Behavioral Observation Profile of the RICE-R (see Figure 14-2) or (2) an overall rating of moderate or mild-to-moderate on the RIC Rating for Cognitive-Communicative Deficits in Right Hemisphere Dysfunction (see Table 14-2).

This group should be held a minimum of twice a week for an hour. Group size may be larger for this group

Behavioral Observation Profile: Rating Scale

	1	2	3	4
Attention	Inattentive (attentive 0%–30% of the time)	Attentive some of the time (31%–60% of the time)	Usually attentive (61%–90% of the time)	Fully attentive (more than 90% of the time)
Awareness of illness	Denies illness or hemiplegia	Aware of illness and/or some major limitations	Aware of some subtle problems but not all	Fully aware
Orientation to person	Does not recognize family or friends	Recognizes highly familiar people	Recognizes some less familiar people but not all	Oriented
Orientation to place	Unaware of present location	Passive orientation to place but cannot find way around environment	Inconsistently finds way around the environment	Oriented
Orientation to time	Unaware of date, time, season	Aware of gross time periods (e.g., season and month) but not specific times (e.g., date, day of the week)	Aware of specific times and inconsistently monitors the passage of time	Oriented
Memory for daily events	Unable to remember any daily events	Remembers some daily events but not all	Remembers most daily events	Remembers all important daily events

Total Score: _____ / 24

FIGURE 14-2.
Behavioral Observation Profile of the RIC Evaluation of Communication Problems in Right Hemisphere Dysfunction–Revised. (Reprinted from AS Halper, LR Cherney, MS Burns [eds]. Clinical Management of Right Hemisphere Dysfunction [2nd ed]. Gaithersburg, MD: Aspen Publishers, 1996; used with permission.)

because patients are at a higher level; optimum size is four to eight patients.

Table 14-4 presents goals, activities, and variables manipulated and measured for each skill that is stressed in the high-level cognitive group. Although this table lists the goals and activities separately, they are often worked on simultaneously. For example, consider the task of retelling a current event from a radio or television newscast. Taking notes can be used as a compensatory memory strategy to remember key information or as a means of improving organizational skills to sequence the order of events. For some patients, it may serve both purposes.

Another example is the patient who has difficulty organizing the day. First, he or she needs to remember what activities should be accomplished during the day. An effective compensatory memory strategy, such as a "to-do" list, may be necessary. Next, the patient should sequence and prioritize the day's activities. Finally, alternatives to the scheduled activities should be considered in case of unforeseen changes. The group participants can help each other evaluate the effectiveness of the compensatory strategy, identify time constraints, and propose alternate schedules.

LIFE SKILLS GROUP

This group is designed to help patients use community resources, such as stores, transportation, and recreational

TABLE 14-2.
Rehabilitation Institute of Chicago Rating for Cognitive-Communicative Disorders in Right Hemisphere Damage

Minimal impairment	The patient communicates in a full range of contexts, although subtle deficits in integrative skills persist.
Mild impairment	The patient appears to communicate adequately in most situations, but specific impairments become apparent in distracting settings or through structured assessment.
Mild-to-moderate impairment	The patient has generally accurate and appropriate communication in most contexts but continues to show problems with attention, orientation, perception, integration, and pragmatics.
Moderate impairment	The patient has functional communication in simple familiar contexts, responding appropriately to most simple stimuli, but continues to show problems with attention, orientation, perception, integration, and pragmatics.
Moderate-to-severe impairment	The patient has marked deficits in attention, orientation, perception, or pragmatics but responds appropriately to some simple stimuli.
Severe impairment	The patient has severe deficits in attention, orientation, perception, and pragmatics and rarely responds appropriately to stimuli.

facilities. It extends the goals of the high-level cognitive group into the community by providing participants with an opportunity to apply their learned compensatory techniques to community situations. Skills that may be stressed in this group are these:

- Planning, organizing, and carrying out community activities
- Responding to everyday problem situations that arise
- Using self-monitoring strategies to make appropriate adaptations

Patients must meet both of the following criteria for admission to this group: (1) an overall rating of mild on the RIC Rating for Cognitive-Communicative Deficits in Right Hemisphere Dysfunction (see Table 14-2) and (2) a goal of community re-entry for vocational or avocation pursuits. Ideally, such a group should be offered through a comprehensive day rehabilitation program but should be open to other outpatients, who may not be eligible for day rehabilitation because they require only speech-language pathology services.

This group should be an interdisciplinary group. Typically, two therapists from the following disciplines facilitate the group depending on its size: occupational therapy, physical therapy, speech-language pathology, and therapeutic recreation. The group meets twice a week. During the first meeting, which lasts 1.0–1.5 hours, activities and outings are planned. In addition, assignments are given that are consistent with each patient's individual goals to facilitate the implementation of the activity. During the second meeting, which lasts 2–4 hours depending on the activity, members of the group participate in the activity. An evaluation of the activity with recommendations and modifications for goals of future activities is an integral part of this second session. In our experience, four to six group members are optimal.

Table 14-5 presents samples of three community activities: going to a restaurant, going shopping, and going on a sightseeing tour. It illustrates how components of each activity are addressed for each goal.

PRAGMATICS GROUP

Disturbances of pragmatics in patients with right hemisphere damage may occur in any of three contexts: (1) extralinguistic, (2) paralinguistic, or (3) linguistic [3]. Extralinguistic problems occur in nonverbal behaviors, such as gestures, body posture, eye contact, and facial expression. The paralinguistic problems are reflected in intonation and prosody. Linguistic deficits occur in the patient's discourse, such as conversation and storytelling. The treatment of pragmatic problems often can be more effective in group situations, where more natural interactions can occur.

The pragmatics group focuses on increasing awareness of extralinguistic, paralinguistic, and linguistic contexts and facilitating appropriate social interactions in a group situation. Skills stressed include these:

- Nonverbal communication skills (intonation, facial expression, eye contact, gestures, proxemics)
- Verbal communication skills (conversation initiation, turn taking, topic maintenance, presupposition, referencing skills)
- Response length
- Informational completeness

This group is appropriate for a variety of levels of care as well as different severity levels of cognitive-communicative problems. Therefore, activities may range from improving basic skills, such as maintaining eye contact with the speaker and using appropriate greetings, to advanced skills, such as acting appropriately in a job interview situation or at a social gathering.

There are no specific criteria for admission to this group because it spans a variety of severity levels. On admission, patients are rated on the Pragmatic Communication Skills Rating Scale of the RICE-R (Figure 14-3). This score helps group patients homogeneously, serves as a baseline for improvement, and targets areas of deficit for treatment.

The frequency with which the pragmatics group is held depends on the level of care and the severity of the impairment, but it should be held at least twice a week. Typically, group size varies from four to six members, regardless of the level of care. It is often helpful to include family members as participants in the group so that they can learn and practice skills to help them become more effective communication partners.

TABLE 14-3.
Orientation Group

Skill	Goal	Variables Manipulated or Measured	Activities
Sustained and selective attention	Patient will use sustained or selective attention for ____ minutes to an auditory or visual stimuli (e.g., instructions, daily schedule, conversation) in a _____- (e.g., structured, dining room, activities room, physical therapy gym) environment	Length Modality Time Introduction of distracters Environment Number and type of cues	Reading a menu (hospital, local restaurant) Reading daily or weekly schedule Participating in a simple conversation about the immediate environment Following or giving instructions Copying or tracing
Attention to left side of space	Patient demonstrates attention to the left side of space for ____ minutes during a _____ task (e.g., object location task, reading, writing, simple route finding) in a _____ (e.g., structured, dining room, activities room, physical therapy gym) environment	Type of stimulus (e.g., objects, letters, words) Size of stimulus Size of environment (e.g., tabletop vs. entire room) Familiarity of environment Type and number of cues	Selecting items from a vending machine Following a simple route Scanning and tracking for designated functional information (e.g., schedule, calendar, grocery or to-do list, menu) Selecting specific information in a newspaper (e.g., date, name, headline)
Remembering personal biographic information	Consistent expression of personal information of _____ pieces of information during simple conversation	Familiarity of information Length of information Self-initiated versus response to questions Type and number of cues	Sharing family photographs Reviewing information sheets about themselves
Perception of environmental cues	Consistent ability to express _____ orientation (e.g., time, place) information using environmental cues	Familiarity of environment Type and number of cues	Routine observation of the environment to determine time (e.g., dark vs. light, snow vs. green grass) and place (e.g., white coats and stethoscope to indicate hospital; stove and refrigerator to indicate kitchen)
Using simple compensatory strategies to retain orientation information	Comprehension and expression of orientation (e.g., time, place, person) information using an external compensatory strategy	Type of compensatory device (e.g., watch, schedule, calendar, simple memory book) Amount of information to be retained Familiarity of information	Routinely review sections of external compensatory device Question-and-answer format to facilitate use of external compensatory device

Table 14-6 lists activities appropriate for specific goals. In general, there is a recommended sequence of treatment procedures for awareness and use of pragmatic skills. Awareness of deficit areas is developed through the use of scripts, then videotapes of others, and finally, videotapes of the patient. Practicing appropriate pragmatic skills should occur first in structured conversation or other discourse activities, then role-playing, and finally in real-life situations.

COMMON ELEMENTS ACROSS GROUPS

Certain elements are common to all these groups: referral procedures, evaluating the group's effectiveness, and discharge criteria. On referral for speech-language pathology services, patients are assigned a primary clinician, who is responsible for completing the initial evaluation and treatment plan. After the evaluation or at any point in the treat-

ment process, the primary clinician may determine the need for a specific group and make an appropriate referral.

Figure 14-4 includes a copy of a referral/update form. The primary clinician is responsible for identifying the appropriate group, delineating initial group treatment goals in collaboration with the patient, and completing the cognitive-communicative checklist. This checklist includes overall severity as determined by the RIC Rating Scale for Cognitive-Communicative Disorders in Right Hemisphere Damage (see Table 14-2), predominant characteristics, and functional status for auditory comprehension, oral expression, reading comprehension, and written expression. The group clinician indicates the date the goal was met and returns the form to the primary clinician for updating. If the patient is being seen only in group, the group speech-language pathologist assumes the role of the primary clinician and updates the goals accordingly.

Although the clinician is treating the cognitive problems underlying communication breakdown, goals must focus on

TABLE 14-4.
High-Level Cognitive Group

Skill	Goal	Variables Manipulated or Measured	Activities
Maximizing effective use of compensatory memory strategies	Patient will demonstrate consistent comprehension and expression of _____ (type of information: daily activities, current events) in a ____-minute conversation using compensatory strategies (e.g., memory book, mnemonic)	Type of compensatory strategy (This must be carefully selected with the patient, taking into consideration such factors as severity of impairment, communication needs, and discharge environment.) Length of information Length of time material needs to be retained Introduction of distracters Number and type of cues	Listening to weather, traffic, sports, or stock market reports Listening, reading, or watching a news broadcast Taking a telephone message Listening for the daily lottery numbers Remembering a new acquaintance's name and other significant information about that person Remembering instructions for taking medications Remembering directions to a destination
Organizing, sequencing, and prioritizing information	Patient will demonstrate consistent organization of information in _____ (e.g., conversational speech, narrative discourse, written material) for _____ (e.g., educational, vocational, avocational) purposes	Length of information Complexity of information Stimulus modality Response modality (written, oral) Number and type of cues	Telling a joke Retelling a story Telling a personal experience Giving directions (e.g., daily procedures such as making a bed, directions to get to a specified location) Retelling a current event from a radio or television newscast Developing a to-do list for a designated activity or for a specified period Listening to a lecture, taking notes, and discussing Prioritizing information (e.g., determining how to spend a limited amount of money, prioritizing running errands, prioritizing weekend activities given time limitations, prioritizing which bills to pay given specific interest rates or limited cash)
Facilitating functional problem solving	Patient will demonstrate consistent problem solving for comprehension and expression of _____ (e.g., everyday situations) for _____ (e.g., educational, vocational, avocational) purposes	Familiarity of the situation Complexity of the situation Number of potential solutions available Number of alternative solutions requested	Discussing solutions to emergency situations (e.g., fires, accidents, illness) Discussing solutions and their consequences to everyday situations (e.g., finding a job, choosing health care providers, choosing your bank) Discussing inconsistencies in a story, joke, or conversation Expressing opinions on controversial issues

communication. Many third-party payers do not reimburse for speech-language pathology services that focus on the rehabilitation of cognitive deficits. Therefore, the clinician must reformulate goals using terminology that is consistent with a communication problem rather than a cognitive-communicative problem. Emphasis should be placed on using terms such as *comprehension* and *expression* of auditory and written language. Table 14-7 provides examples of how to change cognitive goals to communication goals.

Group treatment may be offered in lieu of or as a supplement to individual treatment. Individuals enrolled in any of the groups must demonstrate continued potential for improvement in functional communication skills to receive reimbursement. It is important that the progress of each patient is monitored carefully to ensure that patients are benefiting appropriately from group treatment. Figure 14-5 provides two alternative forms for documenting patient performance during group treatment. One form allows the clinician to document performance over time for an individual patient. A sample log from the orientation group is provided. The other form allows the clinician to document the performance of all the group participants on a specific day.

TABLE 14-5.
Life Skills Group

Activity	Planning, Organizing, Sequencing, and Prioritizing Community Activities	Maximizing Effective Use of Compensatory Strategies for Memory Impairment during a Community Activity	Maximizing Effective Use of Compensatory Strategies for Left-Sided Neglect during a Community Activity	Comprehension and Use of Appropriate Pragmatic Skills in Community Activities	Facilitating Functional Problem Solving during a Community Activity
			Goal		
Going to a restaurant	Deciding on a restaurant based on type of food, cost, and location; Determining location of restaurant and what type of transportation is needed; Determining date and time all members can go to restaurant; Making a reservation	Remembering verbally presented specials of the day using strategies practiced in the high-level cognitive group; Remembering each person's order; Remembering items to be ordered after the menu is closed; Remembering the cost of the items ordered	Scanning menu items and cost	Conversing with other group members; Interacting and giving orders to restaurant help	Making last-minute changes to plans (e.g., cannot walk to restaurant because of inclement weather, what to do if one person is late, what to do if one person does not have enough money); Determining what you ordered based on monetary and dietary restrictions
Going shopping	Determining what you need to buy; Determining which stores carry the items you need; Selecting stores to go to based on location, availability of items, and cost; Determining what type of transportation is needed; Prioritizing which items need to be purchased first; Determining who is responsible for purchasing specific items; if appropriate, break into smaller groups or pairs based on criteria defined by group (e.g., time restrictions, skills of group members)	Remembering what stores you need to go to and what items must be purchased using strategies practiced in higher-level cognitive group; Remembering where and what time to meet at end of community trip	Scanning store aisles for specific items	Requesting information from store help	Making last-minute changes to plans (e.g., cannot walk to mall because of inclement weather, what to do if one person is late, what to do if one person does not have enough money or must purchase an extra item)
Sightseeing tour	Deciding on the sites to be visited; Determining locations of these sites, order in which sites will be visited based on location, route, and type of transportation needed; Determining what exhibits at a site will be visited; Determining dates and times members can go on sightseeing tour and how long will be spent at each site; Determining cost of visits	Remembering specific information gained during the visit for later discussion with group members; Remembering where and what time to meet at end of the visit to each site	Scanning a brochure that describes the site; Following a map of the site, if applicable; Scanning exhibits for predetermined items; Finding and following signs to exhibits	Requesting information about the location of exhibits	Making last-minute changes to plans (e.g., when you arrive the site is closed, or there is a long line to get in)

Pragmatic Communication Skills: Rating Scale

NONVERBAL COMMUNICATION

	1	2	3	4
Intonation	Flat/monotone or inappropriate	Limited or inconsistently appropriate	Appropriate intonation most of the time	Appropriate
Facial expression	Absent or inappropriate	Limited or inconsistently appropriate	Appropriate facial expression most of the time	Appropriate
Eye contact	Cannot establish eye contact	Needs cues to maintain eye contact	Maintains and uses eye contact appropriately most of the time; minimal cues may be needed	Appropriate
Gestures and proxemics	Absent or inappropriate	Limited or inconsistently appropriate	Uses gestures and proxemics appropriately most of the time	Appropriate

VERBAL COMMUNICATION

	1	2	3	4
Conversation initiation	Inappropriate or does not initiate	Limited or inconsistently appropriate initiation	Initiates conversation appropriately most of the time	Appropriate
Turn taking	Unaware of turn-taking signals	Inconsistently responsive to signals	Uses and responds to turn-taking signals appropriately most of the time	Appropriate

continues

FIGURE 14-3.
Pragmatic Communication Skills Rating Scale of the RIC Evaluation of Communication Problems in Right Hemisphere Dysfunction–Revised. (Reprinted from AS Halper, LR Cherney, MS Burns [eds]. Clinical Management of Right Hemisphere Dysfunction [2nd ed]. Gaithersburg, MD: Aspen Publishers, 1996; used with permission.)

Topic maintenance	1 Absent or inappropriate topic maintenance (Maintains topic less than 50% of the time)	2 Maintains topic some of the time (50%–75% of the time)	3 Maintains topic most of the time (76%–90% of the time)	4 Maintains topic (more than 90% of the time)
Response length (Circle on scale whether patient produces verbose or short utterances)	1 Responses are verbose or inappropriately short (more than 50% of the time)	2 Responses are inconsistently verbose or inappropriately short (25%–49% of the time)	3 Appropriate response length most of the time (inappropriate only 10%–24% of the time)	4 Appropriate response length (more than 90% of the time)
Presupposition	1 Presupposes too much and/or too little (more than 50% of the time)	2 Presupposes too much and/or too little some of the time (25%–49% of the time)	3 Occasionally presupposes too much and/or too little (10%–24% of the time)	4 Appropriate (more than 90% of the time)
Referencing skills	1 Inappropriate referencing (more than 50% of the time)	2 Inappropriate referencing some of the time (25%–49% of the time)	3 Occasional inappropriate referencing (10%–24% of the time)	4 Appropriate referencing (more than 90% of the time)

Total Score: _____ / 40

Narrative Discourse—Completeness

The following severity levels are based on the Story Retelling-Immediate Subtest of the *Arizona Battery for Communication Disorders of Dementia* by K.A. Bayles, C.K. Tomoeda, Canyonlands Publishing, Inc., Tucson, AZ (1991). This task has a maximum of 17 information units for completeness.

Completeness	Severe ≤ 9 informational units	Moderate 10–12 informational units	Mild 13–14 informational units	Normal ≥ 15 informational units

FIGURE 14-3. *Continued.*

TABLE 14-6.
Pragmatics Group

Skill	Goal	Variables Manipulated or Measured	Activities
Comprehension and use of nonverbal pragmatic skills	Patient demonstrates consistent comprehension and use of _____ (e.g., facial expressions, intonation, eye contact, gestures, proxemics) in a ____-minute conversation	Familiarity of the context Number of nonverbal features focused on at a given time Number and type of cues	Viewing of videotape of self or others Identifying emotional intent of photographs of people Role-playing specific situations Engaging in a conversation
Improvement of turn-taking skills	Patient demonstrates appropriate use of turn-taking skills in a ____-minute conversation	Familiarity of topic Familiarity of context Familiarity with participants Number of participants Type and number of cues	Identifying conversational turns from a script or videotape Role-playing specific situations Engaging in a conversation
Improvement of topic initiation and maintenance	Patient demonstrates appropriate initiation, maintenance, and shifting of topic in a ____-minute _____ (discourse type: e.g., conversation, narrative story, procedure)	Familiarity of topic Familiarity of context Number of participants Number of changes in topic Type and number of cues	Identifying instances of topic initiation, maintenance and change from a script or videotape Role-playing specific situations Engaging in a conversation Providing directions Giving a lecture Telling a story or personal experience
Increase meaningfulness of informational content	Patient consistently uses meaningful information in a ____-minute _____ (discourse type: e.g., conversation, narrative story, procedure)	Familiarity of topic Familiarity of context Number of participants Type and number of cues	Identifying instances of meaningful and nonmeaningful information from a script or videotape Engaging in a conversation Providing directions Telling a story or personal experience Making a telephone call Barrier tasks
Improvement of cohesion	Patient demonstrates appropriate use of _____ (e.g., pronouns, conjunctions) in a ____-minute _____ (discourse type: e.g., conversation, narrative story, procedure)	Number of potential referents Familiarity with participants Familiarity of context Type and number of cues	Identifying instances of cohesion from a script or videotape Barrier tasks Giving directions Retelling a story or personal experience

It is difficult to develop predetermined discharge criteria because of the variety of factors that must be considered, such as discharge placement, patient and caregiver goals, severity of impairment, and third-party payer limitations. In general, patients are discharged from group treatment when individual goals are achieved or group goals no longer meet the patient's needs. When the patient is discharged from group treatment, the primary clinician or group clinician should ask the patient to fill out the patient satisfaction questionnaire provided in Figure 14-6. If the patient is unable to complete the form independently, the spouse or another clinician on staff should interview the patient using these questions. The patient's responses and suggestions from the survey are shared with the group clinician. Appropriate recommendations are incorporated into the group, and any other required actions are taken.

This chapter has focused on types of groups and associated goals and group activities for treatment of patients with right hemisphere damage across varying levels of care. There is a paucity of information in the literature on group treatment for this population, and studies are needed to determine the efficacy of group treatment techniques. Although we believe that group treatment is an appropriate means of delivering patient care, this chapter is based on clinical experience without supporting data. Nevertheless, group treatment does allow a facility to use staff more efficiently, deliver patient care at a lower cost, and provide treatment in a supportive environment.

GROUP REFERRAL/UPDATE FORM

Patient Name_____ Med. Record #_____

_____Orientation Group   _____Life Skills Group
_____High-Level Cognitive Group   _____Pragmatics Group

PLEASE COMPLETE ATTACHED CHECKLIST AT TIME OF INITIAL REFERRAL.

GOAL	DATE GOAL MET

Clinician_____Date_____

FIGURE 14-4.
Group referral/update form.

COGNITIVE COMMUNICATIVE PROBLEMS SECONDARY TO RIGHT HEMISPHERE DAMAGE

OVERALL SEVERITY
___Minimal   ___ Mild   ___Mild-to-Moderate   ___Moderate
___Moderate-to-Severe   ___Severe

PREDOMINANT CHARACTERISTICS

___Impaired Attention
   ___Sustained attention
   ___Selective attention
   ___Shifting attention
   ___Divided attention
___Distractibility
___Impulsivity
___Left Unilateral Neglect
___Disorientation
   ___Time
   ___Place
   ___Person
___Impaired Visual Perception
___Impaired Memory
   ___Encoding
   ___Storage
   ___Retrieval

___Impaired Pragmatics
   ___Intonation
   ___Facial Expression
   ___Eye Contact
   ___Gestures/Proxemics
   ___Conversational Initiation
   ___Turn-taking
   ___Topic Maintenance
   ___Presupposition
   ___Referencing
   ___Informational Content
   ___Informational
      Completeness
___Impaired Organization
___Impaired Reasoning
___Impaired Problem
   Solving/Judgment

FUNCTIONAL STATUS
Auditory Comprehension: Understands
___Brief statements about immediate environment
___Simple conversation about daily activities and needs
___Simple conversation about variety of topics
___Most complex or abstract conversation
___All complex or abstract conversation

Oral Expression: Discusses
___Basic needs
___Daily activities and ideas
___A variety of topics
___Most complex or abstract ideas
___All complex or abstract ideas

Patient Name_____

COMPLETE IF APPLICABLE

Reading Comprehension: Reading
___Nonfunctional
___Single words
___Phrase length material
___Single sentence
___Simple paragraph
___Several related paragraphs
___Everyday adult-level material
___Most complex or abstract material
___All complex or abstract material
___At premorbid level

Written Expression: Writing (Check level and content)
___Nonfunctional
___Single words
___Phrases
___Sentences
___Paragraphs

___Basic needs
___Daily activities and ideas
___A variety of topics
___Most complex or abstract ideas
___All complex or abstract ideas

Please add any pertinent comments:

FIGURE 14-4. *Continued*

TABLE 14-7.
Rewriting Cognition Goals

	Cognitive Goal	*Rewritten Communication Goal*
Long-term goal	Independently use a memory book to recall daily activities	Consistent comprehension and expression of daily activities in a 15- to 20-minute conversation using a memory book
Short-term goal	(1) 80% accuracy locating requested information from the memory book	(1) 80% accurate reading comprehension of requested information from the memory book
	(2) Accurate documentation of two activities in the memory book	(2) Accurate written expression of two sentences to record daily activities in the memory book
Long-term goal	Consistent retention of information from a 15-minute conversation using self-cueing strategies	Consistent comprehension and expression of information from a 15-minute conversation using self-cueing strategies
Short-term goal	(1) Recall of a three-part message after 15 minutes using compensatory strategies	(1) Accurate expression of a three-part message after 15 minutes using compensatory strategies
	(2) Recall of two treatment activities at the end of 15 minutes	(2) Verbal description of two treatment activities at the end of 15 minutes
Long-term goal	Consistent ability to provide three solutions to functional daily living situations	Consistent ability to express three solutions to functional daily living situations
Short-term goal	(1) 80% accuracy providing one to two solutions to a given problem	(1) 80% accuracy verbally describing one to two solutions to a given problem
	(2) 80% accurate identification of the most appropriate solution to a given problem from a choice of three	(2) Verbal explanation of the most appropriate solution to a given problem 80% of the time
	(3) 80% accuracy solving a four-element deductive problem	(3) 80% accurate reading comprehension of a four-element problem solving task
Long-term goal	Consistent ability to sustain attention to all activities during a 30-minute session	Consistent ability to comprehend all conversation during a 30-minute conversation
Short-term goal	(1) 80% accuracy identifying a target item in a 5-minute auditory vigilance task	(1) 80% accurate comprehension and identification of a target word in a 5-minute auditory task
	(2) Consistent attention to a 5-minute conversation with less than three redirections	(2) Consistent comprehension of a 5-minute conversation with less than three redirections
Long-term goal	Consistent orientation to time, place, and person	Consistent ability to express time, place, and person orientation information
Short-term goal	(1) Consistent orientation to time (day, date, time) using environmental cues	(1) Consistent ability to express time (day, date, time) using environmental cues
	(2) 80% accuracy finding a designated location using environmental signs	(2) 80% reading comprehension of environmental signs to locate a designated place
Long-term goal	Consistent sequencing of 10 pieces of information in a complex planning task	Consistent ability to verbally express 10 steps in the correct sequence to complete a complex task
Short-term goal	(1) Identification of four steps to complete a simple task	(1) Consistent ability to verbally express four steps in the correct sequence to complete a simple task
	(2) 80% accuracy sequencing five written sentences	(2) 80% accurate comprehension and sequencing five written sentences

Date: _____   Clinician: _____

__X__ Orientation group   _____ Life skills group

_____ High-level cognitive group   _____ Pragmatics group

Patient

Activity	*JR*	*TW*	*FC*	*KL*
Scanning calendar for 5 major holidays and days they fall on	Identified 2 with verbal cues	Identified 1 with verbal cues	Identified 4 with verbal cues	Identified 3 with verbal cues
Scanning picture of hospital vending machine for potato chips	Identified 2 of 6 with verbal cues	Identified 3 of 6 with verbal and visual (red line) cues	Identified 4 of 6 with verbal cues	Identified 3 of 6 with verbal cues

Patient name: _____   Medical record no.: _____

Clinician: _____

__X__ Orientation group   _____ Life skills group

_____ High-level cognitive group   _____ Pragmatics group

Response

Activity	*8/11/97*	*8/12/97*	*8/13/97*	*8/14/97*	*8/15/97*
Scanning calendar for 5 major holidays and days they fall on in 1998	Identified 3 with verbal cues	Identified 5 with verbal cues	Identified 5 with no cues		
Scanning picture of hospital vending machine for potato chips	Identified 3 of 6 with verbal and visual (red line) cues	Identified 3 of 6 with verbal cues	Identified 4 of 6 with verbal cues	Identified 6 of 6 with verbal cues	
Scanning hospital vending machine for potato chips				Identified 3 of 6 with verbal and gestural cues	Identified 4 of 6 with verbal and gestural cues

FIGURE 14-5.
Group treatment log.

Patient name: _____   Medical record no.: _____

Interviewer: _____   Date: _____

____ **Orientation group**   ____ **Life skills group**

____ **High-level cognitive group**   ____ **Pragmatics group**

1. How satisfied were you with the group treatment?

____Very satisfied   ____ Satisfied   ____ Not satisfied

2. What did you work on in group?

3. What activities were helpful?

4. What activities were not helpful?

5. Did you get to know the other members of the group?   ____ Yes ____ No

6. Do you feel you received enough attention in the group? ____ Yes ____ No

7. What suggestions do you have to improve the group?

FIGURE 14-6.
Patient satisfaction questionnaire.

REFERENCES

1. American Speech-Language-Hearing Association. The role of speech-language pathologists in the habilitation and rehabilitation of cognitively impaired adults: a report of the subcommittee on language. ASHA 1987;29:53–55.
2. Cherney LR, Halper AS. A Conceptual Framework for the Evalua-
tion and Treatment of Communication Problems Associated with Right Hemisphere Damage. In AS Halper, LR Cherney, MS Burns (eds), Clinical Management of Right Hemisphere Dysfunction (2nd ed). Gaithersburg, MD: Aspen Publishers, 1996;21–29.
3. Davis GA. Pragmatics and Treatment. In R Chapey (ed), Language Intervention Strategies in Adult Aphasia (2nd ed). Baltimore: Williams & Wilkins, 1986.

SECTION IV

Traumatic Brain Injury

CHAPTER FIFTEEN

Traumatic Brain Injury: Cognitive-Communicative Needs and Early Intervention

Rita J. Gillis

CHARACTERISTICS OF TRAUMATIC BRAIN INJURY

Before beginning a discussion about group therapy for people who have sustained a traumatic brain injury (TBI), it is important to differentiate this population from other populations discussed in this text. First, terminology is still not widely agreed on in the field of neurorehabilitation. A variety of terms have been used to refer to the population addressed in this chapter, including *closed head injury, closed head trauma, nonfocal brain damage,* and *acquired brain damage or injury.* The use of the term *TBI* has been advocated to indicate that there has been a brain injury, whereas the term *head injury* includes skull fractures, scalp lacerations, and facial injuries, with or without injury to the brain. Because *head injury* does not identify the structure of primary concern when there has been trauma to the head, TBI is preferred for its greater specificity. It differentiates brain damage that occurs as a result of trauma from that which occurs secondary to other conditions, such as cerebrovascular disease, tumor, or infection.

TBI technically refers to both penetrating and nonpenetrating injuries that result in brain damage attributable to external forces. Generally, in medical literature, TBI refers to nonpenetrating injuries, most often resulting from motor vehicle accidents and violent crimes. Here, and in general use, TBI refers to injuries that result in diffuse axonal injury (DAI), which is the primary differentiating characteristic. (The scope of this text precludes a detailed discussion of DAI. For an introductory review of the mechanisms of DAI and the associated pathophysiology, see Gillis and Pierce [1] and Gennarelli [2].)

The frontal lobes and temporal poles are highly susceptible to damage from the bony prominences of the skull after TBI. Frontal lobe impairment, particularly in prefrontal regions, and the association with decreased functioning in executive skills are significant contributing factors to the communication impairment observed in this population. It is the widespread, diffuse nature of the brain damage, often paired with focal lesions, that results in the great diversity of impairment that confronts clinicians. Recovery of physical and cognitive abilities after TBI, in contrast to recovery after stroke, occurs at a highly variable rate, often with dramatic changes. As such, assessment and treatment must be conducted with a great deal of flexibility and sensitivity to changes in the individual's abilities.

It is well recognized today that communication impairment after TBI is not the same as that which results from other types of acquired brain damage, such as stroke. Although aphasia may accompany TBI, it is rarely the predominant feature [3]. Many terms have been used to describe the nature of communication impairment that accompanies TBI. The term used commonly today is *cognitive-communicative impairment,* as proposed by the American Speech-Language-Hearing Association. The term reflects the integrated aspects of cognition and communication and the predominant cognitive component of the impairment.

STAGES OF RECOVERY

The Rancho Los Amigos Levels of Cognitive Functioning (LOCF) [4] scale has proved to be a useful tool in the field of TBI rehabilitation, providing clinicians from several disciplines with a common vocabulary to discuss cognitive recovery from TBI. It has been reprinted in numerous texts [5–7] available to speech-language pathologists and is only summarized here. The scale has become such a standard observation tool in rehabilitation settings that when clinicians discuss *early, middle,* and *late* stages of recovery [8], they are usually referring to the LOCF, as I do here. Levels I, II, and III refer to early periods of recovery, as identified by the LOCF, in which responsiveness to the environment is key. Group therapy for the early stages of recovery is discussed briefly in this chapter, but the use of a group format at this stage is questionable. Levels IV, V, and VI reflect an increase in responsiveness and orientation, and at this point group therapy is sometimes more appropriate. At the last two levels, VII and VIII, confusion has resolved, and people are more purposeful in their behavior than before. In these stages of recovery, group therapy can be very effective in addressing cognitive-communicative needs. These levels are provided as a guideline for cognitive functioning at different stages of recovery, but many people exhibit a range of behaviors from different levels simultaneously [8].

Problems in arousal and attention, which are particularly noteworthy soon after regaining consciousness, are characteristic of TBI. The confusion and disorientation witnessed in the early stages of recovery are indices of disordered attention. Post-traumatic amnesia (PTA) is a symptom of the difficulty people experience in information processing after TBI and is defined as the inability to remember information after the injury. People are thought to have recovered from PTA when they remember new information on a day-to-day or continuous basis. PTA is of particular concern to clinicians and should be monitored daily. As long as people are experiencing PTA, new learning is greatly reduced, if it occurs at all.

As people progress, they are able to process information more effectively and can be oriented, which leads to less confusion. However, many people with TBI remain "confusable" [8,9] and can be easily overloaded with information. Slowed and inefficient information processing is cited frequently as a major sequela of TBI [10–12]. As such, people may experience difficulty processing auditory and visual information, particularly as length and complexity increase. Memory impairment is almost always reviewed in the literature as a major long-term, neurobehavioral consequence of TBI [13]. Problems related to memory failure may occur as a result of attentional limitations or difficulty with encoding, storage, and retrieval. Many people have difficulty retaining information from day to day, thereby posing a unique challenge to clinicians.

Inefficient word recall and disorganized verbal output also may be observed at various stages and as a long-term impairment. In addition to these problems in learning and relaying information, which are reviewed extensively in the literature, people with TBI have a variety of problems related to poor executive control [14]. Problems in executive control can be observed as difficulty in solving problems, fragmentation or disorganization of actions, poor monitoring of performance and output, and a limited awareness of strengths and weaknesses. In social or conversational situations, people may have difficulty in monitoring verbal output, anticipating responses of others, initiating conversations or taking turns, following nonverbal signs, monitoring vocal tone and intensity, and responding to and using a variety of speech acts. Little research has been done in this area, particularly in the field of speech-language pathology, yet it is well documented in outcome studies [15–17] that one of the greatest difficulties people have in successfully resuming productive and enjoyable lifestyles is poor psychosocial skills.

This is only a brief overview of the nature of cognitive-communicative impairment after TBI. It does not provide enough depth to guide clinicians new to the field. The reader is referred to other sources [1,18–24] for detailed discussions of those topics.

PHILOSOPHY AND ENTRY CRITERIA

Most would agree that people with TBI are a distinct and diverse group who warrant specialized services. In practice, however, many facilities treat people with other types of acquired brain damage, too. As such, groups may be formed on the basis of cognitive-communicative needs rather than etiology of the impairment. Although a few people with TBI may also have aphasia, perhaps particularly those working with a speech-language pathologist, the extent of cognitive impairment may be such that they should not be grouped with people whose primary need is aphasia therapy. This must be considered on an individual basis, depending on the group dynamics and the people. The differences in age and position in life may make it difficult to plan appropriate long-term goals for a 20-year-old with TBI in a group of clients who are older than 60 years of age. So, although the cognitive-communicative needs of people with TBI are unlikely to be met in groups of people with the predominant impairment of aphasia (or vice versa), there are exceptions.

Unlike many other populations with communication impairments, group therapy is used widely in the field of TBI rehabilitation. (To my knowledge, no studies have examined the differences in effectiveness between individual and group treatment for this population.) In many facilities, group therapy is the only format used. This is partly due to economics, the relative youthfulness of the population and need for social integration, and the fact that many facilities have modeled their programs after those of the New York University (NYU) Medical Center [25] and Presbyterian Hospital in Oklahoma City [9]. The leaders of these programs, Yehuda Ben-Yishay and George Prigatano, respectively, had strong convictions that group interventions were necessary to address the psychosocial needs of people with TBI. Although numerous facilities use group treatment in their rehabilitation programs, to my knowledge these are the only two well-documented *pro-*

grams. However, many clinicians have reported on different types of groups that are used to address a variety of skills, some of which are discussed later. Both programs were outpatient and provided a full or near-full day of mostly group therapies for a specified length of time (e.g., 6 months). They established criteria for entrance into the program as a whole. As an example, participation in the NYU program (hence, in the group therapies) was based on the following conditions [26]:

> independence in ambulation and basic activities of self-care; the ability to engage in reliable two-way verbal communication (i.e., having no more than milder forms of aphasia or dysarthria); the ability to engage in vigorous cognitive and interpersonal remedial "exercises" for several hours a day; a minimum testable IQ of 80 at the point of entry; at least a minimum degree of motivation to attend a rehabilitation program; the absence of blatant, severe, acute psychiatric disturbances; the ability to respond to noncoercive, "social" forms of restraint or disciplines; and a degree of "malleability."

These programs are mentioned because of the influence they have had as models for TBI rehabilitation. Most clinicians do not work in a model program. Today, few rehabilitation facilities have the luxury of admitting a group of clients who begin and end the program at the same time. Clinicians must decide whether groups should be closed or open to new members as patients are admitted to the facility.

Typically, rehabilitation facilities have admission criteria that determine some characteristics of the population receiving treatment. Admission criteria, particularly in outpatient settings, often include a minimal level of cognitive functioning using the LOCF (e.g., clients must be functioning at or above a Rancho level VI). In the current competitive market, however, where many facilities compete for patients, minimal criteria are often used for program admission and may be based more on safety and security issues than on the patient's level of functioning. Therefore, clinicians may want to use criteria for group membership that are more restrictive than the program or facility's admission criteria.

Deaton [27] has suggested the following criteria for group inclusion that are not specific to any particular level of recovery:

1. The specific deficit area addressed by the group should be an area of weakness shared by all group members.

2. Should some group members have difficulty controlling their verbal or physical behavior, enough therapists or other staff members should be available so that no one in the group is injured and so that the group session can continue after interruptions. It is not recommended that people be excluded from all groups based on disruptive or aggressive behavior, because these are common characteristics of people with TBI and can be dealt with effectively in a social context.

3. Should some group members have difficulty with verbal expression, accommodations should be made for

them to express themselves appropriately via written communications, sign language, alphabet board, or augmentative communication devices. Sufficient personnel should be provided to enable efficient communication and to minimize frustration.

These criteria are meant to include a variety of patients across the continuum of care. In an outpatient rehabilitation center, where most people have progressed in their cognitive abilities beyond significant disorientation, confusion, and agitation, more narrow criteria may be desired that include the ability to control aggressive behavior most of the time. Groups in outpatient and transitional settings are apt to be more stable and last for longer periods than are groups formed in an acute medical setting. As such, highly disruptive people, regardless of the number of staff available for supervision, constantly interfere with the goals of the group unless the group is specifically designed to address behavioral problems (i.e., it is a behavioral management group). This type of group may be co-facilitated by a speech-language pathologist if some aspect of improved communication is a goal, but it should be managed by a behavioral specialist, such as a psychologist.

Because of the variability of the population and the type of rehabilitation settings, it is not feasible to provide criteria that are adequate for entrance into all possible groups. For example, a memory group conducted in an acute medical setting for the early stages of recovery would require criteria very different from that of a memory group conducted in a community re-entry setting. An entire text is needed to address the spectrum of TBI rehabilitation. Many groups do not address the needs of the profoundly or mildly injured, people with severe behavioral disorders, or children.

In my opinion, inclusion for group membership is best determined by the needs of the people, the purpose of the group, and the goals of the group. For example, many groups at the community re-entry level require a basic level of communication skills, which might include these abilities: following simple instructions, using at least simple phrases, reading at the simple paragraph level, and participating in therapy sessions 1–2 hours long. For the most part, the group therapy examples provided here require these abilities to meet the goals of the group and use the recommended staff-patient ratios. Chapters 15 and 16 are meant to offer clinicians examples of *some* groups that can be used with the TBI population and should not be seen as comprehensive.

Finally, before moving on to some of the types of groups used in TBI rehabilitation, it is important to distinguish between group therapy and therapy conducted in a group or with a group of people. The distinction is not always easy to make, particularly during the community re-entry phase of rehabilitation. Any number of therapy activities can be conducted with a group of patients that could be effectively carried out individually with a therapist. Therapy provided in this format often has more to do with economics (i.e., it is an efficient use of staff and materials) than with the benefits of group interaction. When conducting therapy with several people at one time, the clinician must weigh the

supportive benefit to clients of being with a group of people with similar needs against other considerations, such as distractions, multiple variables that must be addressed simultaneously, and less of the therapist's time for individual instruction. This is not to say that no benefits other than cost effectiveness pertain to therapy activities conducted with a group of patients. Working in a group of peers can be motivating, may be less threatening than one-to-one therapy, provides an opportunity for socialization, and is more similar to natural social settings than individual therapy, which may promote the generalization of skills. These are benefits when group activities are planned with them in mind. In contrast to working *in a group*, group therapy is used because it is the best format for achieving certain goals. These goals require at least one of the following skills: interaction with peers, group cooperation and teamwork to accomplish a task, modeling of appropriate behaviors (which are a focus of the group), and getting feedback from other members. Because both types of groups are prevalent in TBI rehabilitation, a variety of examples is presented.

ASSESSMENT

Those who have worked in the field of TBI rehabilitation know that traditional aphasia batteries are inadequate to assess the full spectrum of cognitive-communicative impairment. Before deciding to use group therapy to address the cognitive-communicative needs of TBI patients, one must understand the cognitive strengths and weaknesses of each person. Table 15-1 provides an

TABLE 15-1.
Aspects of Cognition to Assess before Group Placement

Attention
    Arousability and lethargy
    Focus and distractibility
    Selective
    Divided
    Sustained
    Controlled and automatic processes
Memory
    Short-term
    Episodic and semantic
    Declarative and procedural
    Prospective
    New learning
    Encoding, storage, and retrieval
Problem solving and reasoning
    Planning and sequencing
    Convergent and divergent thinking
    Deductive reasoning
    Inductive reasoning
    Analogous reasoning
Executive functions or control
    Initiation
    Anticipation and flexibility
    Goal formation
    Self-awareness
    Self-regulation and monitoring
    Inhibition

overview of some areas of cognitive functioning with which clinicians should be familiar before making decisions about group placement. Clinicians need to have a handle on these areas of cognitive functioning through direct testing, observation, and neuropsychological reports, when available.

At one time, aphasia tests and batteries were the only tools available to speech-language pathologists. Today, an arsenal of assessment tools can be used to help clinicians in the diagnostic process. It is assumed that patients receive, or that the clinician has access to, a comprehensive evaluation before group therapy is begun. The nature of the evaluation varies with the stage of recovery.

Although a thorough, formal evaluation is useful, many standard tests simply do not tap the aspects of functioning that are most debilitating in everyday experience. The evaluation setting itself is often so structured that it provides for optimal performance, which is not likely to be reproduced in daily settings. Many of the skills that are addressed effectively in group therapy are also best evaluated in that format, such as initiation of conversation. Although clinicians may find some published scales of behavior (such as social skills or pragmatics) to be useful in monitoring group therapy progress, more often than not clinicians must devise tools tailored to each group.

TYPES OF GROUPS

Early Stages of Recovery

People who are emerging from coma and respond minimally to the environment may benefit from sensory stimulation, which some have suggested can be provided in a group. Before conducting a sensory stimulation group, clinicians should become well acquainted with the literature on coma stimulation, sensory stimulation, and persistent vegetative state. Several critical reviews [28,29] are available to help clinicians examine the benefits and concerns. In some settings, speech-language pathologists may be expected to participate in or lead a sensory stimulation group. A brief discussion is therefore included in this chapter, but clinicians are cautioned to recognize the limitations of group intervention at this level.

Deaton [27] described some of the objectives of a sensory stimulation group: increasing arousal, providing orienting information, identifying and reinforcing responses, and encouraging discrimination between stimuli. The reason for conducting sensory stimulation in a group is largely economic. Because patients are minimally responsive, it is doubtful they could benefit from the responses of peer feedback. Several scales [30,31] can be used to document responsiveness to sensory stimulation. Before beginning therapy, an objective measurement should be taken using a scale. Repeated measures should be taken at least weekly. People who do not demonstrate measurable changes should be discharged after a specified time, such as 2 weeks.

Middle Stages of Recovery

Orientation and Recovery from Post-Traumatic Amnesia
In the middle stages of recovery, people have emerged from coma and respond to their environment, but they are often disoriented and confused and exhibit disorganized thinking. After emergence from coma, PTA is an important variable to monitor. In many settings, this may be done by the speech-language pathologist. The Galveston Orientation and Amnesia Test [32] is commonly used for this purpose and could be administered as part of an orientation group. Corrigan and colleagues [33] have reported on the use of the Group Orientation Monitoring System, which was designed for use in an orientation group conducted at their facility. In the middle stages, decreasing confusion through improved orientation and thought organization is a primary therapeutic goal that can be addressed through orientation, organization, and memory groups, which may go by various names. If stability is maintained, groups in and of themselves can provide important information to clients that can help reduce confusion by imposing structure through regularity and predictability. Additionally, it is important to monitor the recovery from PTA in a systematic, objective manner. Orientation groups can provide clinicians with this opportunity and with the opportunity to assess any negative changes in cognitive function due to medical reasons, such as medication toxicity.

Table 15-2 presents an example of an orientation group. Although many facilities combine orientation and memory book training, in my experience, clients who are disoriented can be overwhelmed, and they become more confused when expected to keep up with and use a note-

TABLE 15-2.
Example of an Orientation Group

Staff-to-patient ratio: 1:4
Frequency: Daily, in AM
Group size: 6–8 (smaller if agitated patients attend)
Goals for group
- Be oriented to person, place, and time
- Identify group members
- Distinguish staff from peers
- Use environmental cues or aids to facilitate orientation
- Recall episodic events
- Use a schedule card to identify next appointment

Suggestions for individual goals: Include percentages for each goal, percentage of all orienting activities, or percentage improvement on a formal measure of orientation (e.g., GOAT).

Variables important to control
- Maintain stability
- Meet in the same room
- Meet at the same time
- Maintain the same staff members
- Follow the same routine for activities
- Place orienting information in the same location
- Maintain form and location of schedule card
- Use activities for episodic recall that are distinctive and do not occur routinely

---

GOAT = Galveston Orientation and Amnesia Test.

book or organizer. A daily journal or memory log with simple entries can be maintained by clinicians to help patients review their day with staff or family members.

Of particular concern to clinicians conducting an orientation group is the highly agitated patient, who may not profit from being in a group and also may interfere dramatically with others' ability to benefit. If patients who are known to become easily agitated are included in the group, it is imperative that there be ample staff available to remove patients to a quiet, nonthreatening setting if they should become highly agitated.

Documentation of progress in an orientation group should always include a formal assessment of orientation and memory, before the initiation of activities and before people are cued to use environmental aids. Once an assessment is made, name tags can be given to group members to aid identification. Calendars and clocks should be visible, and therapy should be conducted in a room with windows. Paper-and-pencil activities are not readily distinguishable from each other; therefore, each session should include some event or activity that can be distinguished from one day to the next. Examples might include identifying different fragrances or smells, making a sculpture from modeling clay, watching a brief news segment and identifying the focus, playing an easy card game, celebrating a birthday, having a guest appear, or taking a walk around the facility.

Ideally, patients should be discharged from the group when all goals have been achieved. If the group is highly variable, however, which is likely given the stage of recovery, some people may be quite disoriented, and others may have difficulty only with episodic recall. The best solution is to have an advanced group, such as a memory group, which can incorporate the goals of the higher-functioning individuals, who otherwise might become frustrated by routine orienting activities. All too often, established groups become holding pens for people, with a justification such as, "It won't hurt her to go through orientation activities." This should be avoided with all groups.

Because orientation affects all therapists' treatment, it is often beneficial to have several team members participate in the group, as long as balance is maintained. It is frequently advantageous to include nursing staff because of their awareness of the preceding evening's events, which might affect some patients' confusion. In theory, this is a good idea, but it is often difficult to achieve in practice, because of the time constraints placed on the nursing staff. With some flexibility from all staff, however, this constraint can be overcome. In an acute care hospital where I was responsible for an orientation group, we moved the group from the first-floor therapy room to a day room on the third-floor bed unit. The group was then close enough to the nursing station so that in the event of a crisis on the floor, any nurse participating in the group was readily available. The attendance of the nursing staff increased dramatically, and overall group communication improved as well.

Groups for Attention and Information Processing
Improving attentional abilities is often included as a goal of an orientation group or a "low-level group," as some [6]

people have called early-intervention groups. Frequently, goals are written in broad terms (e.g., "increase ability to sustain attention in a group setting" or "improve attention to conversation"). The structure and stimulation offered by an orientation group do focus members' attention, and as such, address attention indirectly. However, unless specific goals are set and therapy activities are directed toward attention processes or components of attention, improvement in attention is difficult to assess in any quantitative manner, particularly in a group setting. Additionally, because attention is limited when disorientation is of primary concern, it may be difficult to allow enough time to directly address goals other than orientation goals. Attention is often best addressed through highly structured activities that can be completed within specified periods, such as the Attention Process Training program used by Sohlberg and Mateer [34]. Personal experience suggests that these types of activities are best used in individual therapy, where distractions and the degree of structure can be controlled.

Some aspects of attention can be addressed in a group format at this stage. A number of structured activities lend themselves to a group format, and quantitative measurements, using frequencies or percentages, can be taken. Although it is easy to use groups to address a wide range of skills simultaneously, it is better to address attention specifically rather than attempting to accomplish too many goals with one group. The following example is taken from a team report at a rehabilitation facility that conducted most treatment in groups; unfortunately, it is representative of what many therapists try to accomplish in one group. Goals for the Orientation and Memory Group included these: increase attention, increase orientation to self and facility, increase use of memory notebook, increase awareness of excessive verbalization, improve thought organization, increase quality of verbal exchanges, increase daily recall, and increase social skills. Although a group may benefit many of these areas, it would be difficult to focus on individual needs with such an array of global objectives. Activities that could be used to direct an attention or information-processing group are given in Table 15-3.

The activities suggested in Table 15-3 require selective attention, divided attention, sustained attention, and shifting of attention. They do not rely on recall, and they should not be taken as exercises to increase memory span or to remember increasingly longer bits of information. The goal is to address the initial stages of information processing. Some activities may require more than one aspect of attention, but clinicians should strive to use tasks that do not require multiple skills, particularly for assessment purposes. Any number of variations of these activities can be used, but they should be realistic and simulate information to which the group is likely to attend in everyday experiences. This type of group is particularly well suited to meet the needs of students who will need to perform similar activities and take notes.

Documentation for this type of group can be made easier for therapists by designing forms that patients can complete themselves. This not only provides therapists with objective measurements but also encourages patients

TABLE 15-3.
Example of an Information-Processing Group

Staff-to-patient ratio: 1:4
Frequency: 3–5 times weekly
Group size: 3–6
Goals for group
- Identify auditorily presented stimuli
- Recognize (select) target information, such as telephone numbers, names, descriptions, or instructions in listening exercises
- Take notes to aid in retrieval of information
- Shift attention from one task to another when signaled
- Divide attention between two tasks
- Attend to a sequence of information to complete a task

Suggestions for individual goals: Establish goals for each member based on any or all of the above using frequencies or percentages, depending on individual ability.

Sample activities
Play prerecorded phone messages with names, numbers and instructions. Choose only one target to listen for, such as a name. Instruct members to write the information on a card or piece of paper when they hear it. Rotate around the group to ask for the target. Other members can verify the accuracy of responses.

Read short paragraphs with a name, number, object, color, or some other single bit of information repeated throughout. Have members tally each time the target was heard. The task of reading the paragraph can be rotated among members. Group members verify the number of times the target was heard.

Play prerecorded, short news segments. Alert members to listen for a target piece of information by saying, "This news segment is about a fire. Listen for the city where the fire occurred."

Play prerecorded police communications or other dispatch communications and alert members to listen for a target, such as the name of a suspect, color of clothing, or direction of pursuit.

Play prerecorded broadcasts as above and alert each member to listen for a different piece of information (e.g., one listens for who, another for what, when, where, how, why, and so on).

Give directions to a particular location on a simple map given to each member. Members should mark the location. They can take notes on the directions and then find the location, or they can follow along as the directions are given. The "giving directions task" can be rotated among members if directions are printed.

Have each group member perform some simple task, different from each other, such as a cancellation task. Ring a bell or use some other signal for them to stop the activity and pass it to the next member. The activity can continue until all tasks have been attempted by each member.

to begin to be self-reflective and to monitor their performance and behaviors in a nonthreatening way. Patients should not be expected to be terribly reflective at this stage, but they are apt to receive "hard data" better than verbal feedback from the clinician. Figure 15-1 is an example of a simple form that could be used. After each trial, group members fill in the number of items they correctly detected and the ones they missed. Performance can be discussed as a group, and if someone disagrees with the total number of items presented, the task can be repeated. At the end of the week, members can calculate their overall performance from the form.

Memory and Organization Groups
Memory groups may be found in the acute and post-acute rehabilitation settings for people in the late-middle and late stages of cognitive recovery. Although it may be tempting to design memory groups that use drill exercises

to "practice" recall or encoding, no evidence supports the use of these activities to improve functional memory skills. There is also little evidence to support therapeutic activities designed to practice the use of internal strategies, such as chunking or visual imagery [35]. Although a few single case studies [36] have demonstrated that some patients can be taught to use mnemonics, it is unlikely that any single strategy could be used in a group setting that would meet the needs of each member. Additionally, there is no evidence to suggest that internal memory strategies are used functionally outside of therapy trials. This is not to say that rehearsal and practice do not affect material-specific learning, but only that these activities do not improve overall memory functioning.

Szekeres and colleagues [8,37] and others [6], have stressed the importance of organizing processes to the encoding and retrieval of information and using an indirect approach to memory therapy that focuses on organizing processes: "these processes include analyzing information; identifying relevant perceptual and conceptual features; comparing features and concepts; identifying similarities and differences; classifying and categorizing; sequencing; and integrating information into larger units" [8]. In addition to memory impairment, disorganization of thoughts and actions is of primary concern in the middle stages of recovery. Many activities, from simple to complex, can be conceptualized as organizing activities. Therapy activities at this stage should be designed to develop awareness that information is organized by certain schemes or properties and to identify relationships between objects, events, and people. The goal should be for individuals to eventually impose organizing strategies (either consciously or automatically) that facilitate information processing and access of information. Because organization is involved as an aspect of planning and problem solving, basic organizing processes serve as prerequisite skills to more complex cognitive behaviors that require the integration of skills and information.

ACTIVITIES TO ADDRESS ORGANIZATION. A variety of activities can be used in a group format to address some of the organizing processes discussed above. Organization groups, which often are simply referred to as *cognitive groups*, can easily be adapted to accommodate the needs of late recovery patients by advancing the complexity of the activities used. Therapists can facilitate organized thinking by using a structured procedure, such as a feature analysis guide (discussed by Haarbauer-Krupa and colleagues [37]). These authors have used a printed guide with boxes of predefined categories (groups, action, associations, properties, location, and use) to help patients search through semantic memory to obtain information about a familiar object, event, or person. We know these activities as categorization and verbal association activities. The goal of organization groups is not simply recall or listing, however, but rather to help patients impose order by using a systematic approach to activities. The feature analysis guide or any similar printed guides provide the "concreteness" often needed by patients with TBI. Examples of activities that can be used to address organization are given in Table 15-4.

Name of activity (e.g., listening for a specific item)	Monday (# correct/ # missed)	Tuesday (# correct/ # missed)	Wednesday (# correct/ # missed)	Thursday (# correct/ # missed)	Friday (# correct/ # missed)
Trial 1	e.g., 3/5				
Trial 2					
Trial 3					
Trial 4					
Trial 5					
Name of activity					
Trial 1					
Trial 2					
Trial 3					
Trial 4					
Trial 5					
Name of activity					
Trial 1					
Trial 2					
Trial 3					
Trial 4					
Trial 5					
Name:			**Date:**	**Group:**	

FIGURE 15-1.
Form that patients can use to document performance.

In the late stages of recovery, disorganization and "confusability" may persist, in addition to impaired executive functioning. Groups that address organization at this stage of treatment should incorporate an added dimension that focuses on the patient's self-analysis of organizing principles and reflection on the success or improvement on the process. Although activities can advance in complexity, it is important that they be grounded in functionality or the "real world."

Workbooks with organizational activities abound in our profession, yet many of these activities are not suited to the people we treat. Although it may be easy to list the steps to baking a cake, this is not a realistic activity for a group of young adults with brain injuries, who might have a greater need for learning the steps to using the public transportation system or a fax machine. It is always best to use activities that are relevant to the members of the group, even in simple activities.

MEMORY BOOK TRAINING.   Little evidence supports the direct retraining of memory after TBI, although memory impairment is often a persistent, debilitating consequence. In most

TABLE 15-4.
Types of Activities to Improve Organization

Types of ordering activities
List steps to simple procedural tasks. Have members write steps on cards, list all responses on a board, and discuss the merit of each list in terms of necessary and unnecessary steps.

List steps to procedural tasks (as above), and limit the number of steps. Discuss the steps in terms of essentialness and efficiency.

Give each member a card with a single step to a procedure or activity and have the group sequence the steps.

Types of association activities*
- Identify differences and similarities between items, and discuss the reasoning
- Group items by likeness or function, and discuss the reasoning.
- List items that belong together by function, physical attributes, or some other feature. Accept all possibilities, and then review or discuss the merit of each item.

Other activities to relate to personal or long-term stories
Read or tell a story and ask members to relate some aspect of the story to an event in their personal past. Discuss the personal event, how it relates to the story, and how the "relating" might help to facilitate recall. Test members' recall the next day or next session.

Show pictures of events, actions, or photographs of people and complete task as above, cueing members to purposefully relate the information to something or someone personal.

---

*These activities can be varied by presenting items orally, printed on cards, written on a board, or with pictures or photographs and by using people, events, and objects. Difficulty is increased by abstractness and number.

TABLE 15-5.
Example of a Memory Book Training Group

Staff-to-patient ratio: 1:5
Frequency: Daily, preferably in AM
Group size: 6–8
Primary goal: Use a simple memory book (or organizer) with minimal assistance in a rehabilitation setting.
Subgoals
- To locate information in the memory book; must know sections in book and the information each section contains
- To use a calendar; must know what information is found and placed on the calendar
- To follow a routine schedule (i.e., one with few variations)
- To use a "to-do" list; must know what type of information goes on this list

Advanced goal: Use an organizer of choice as needed for daily activities
Suggestions for individual goals: These goals can be tailored to the individual on a weekly basis, with either percentages or level of cueing or assistance. For example, "John will identify sections in memory book with 75% accuracy."
Examples of book sections
    Autobiographic or emergency information
    Calendar
    Schedule (daily or weekly)
    "To-do" or assignment list
    Diary or journal
    Directions and maps
Examples of questions to direct therapy
    How many sections are in your book?
    What are the sections?
    What type of information can be found in the first section?
    What type of information goes on the calendar?
    What is the autobiographic section for?
    Where can you find a list of things to do?
    What do you write in the journal section?
    What do you do at the end of each task?
    What type of information is under directions?
    Why do you need a directions section?
    Where can you find appointments?

---

treatment settings, memory impairment is addressed through memory book training, which is actually compensation training. Unfortunately, clinicians often think of using a memory book as memory training versus compensation training and fail to take the necessary steps to teach people *how to use* a memory aid, which is crucial to success. Too often, patients with memory disorders are given notebooks, cued to fill in information on a daily basis (often in a group), and are then expected to use them spontaneously. Sohlberg and Mateer [38,39] have referred to the initial stage of memory book training as the *acquisition stage*, in which the individual learns how to use an aid. In their training program, they used a question-and-answer format that included questions similar to those listed in Table 15-5. When people are functioning at similar levels, such as just beginning to learn how to use an aid, memory book training can be carried out effectively in a group setting of a small size. Although each person's choice of organizer or memory notebook may vary, most people benefit by using the sample sections given in Table 15-5. Training should be conducted in a systematic fashion to the point of overlearning. A standard set of questions should be developed and asked each session so that progress can be measured.

When working with memory notebooks, it is important to use simplicity as a guide and not overload the organizer with too many subgroupings, thereby increasing the burden on the individual. Additional headings or dividers can always be added later, as indicated or desired by the individual. A common mistake in programs that do not have tight interdisciplinary programming and team communication is to overload the "to-do" list with assignments from each team member's therapy session. The advantage of the interdisciplinary team approach is that the number of

assignments given to a patient during a particular week can be worked out in advance in team meetings. Thus, the number of assignments can be increased gradually, as the patient learns to use a "to-do" list.

Depending on the composition of the group, it may be necessary to break down the memory book training into a few sections at a time. Some people may be able to use only two or three sections. This must be determined on an individual basis and may not become apparent until the group has met for several sessions. As people become competent in finding information, schedules can have greater variance, and more items can be added to the "to-do" list. In the latter stages of notebook training, people should learn where to look to find out what needs to be done in the future and should be trained to make and keep appointments.

Although memory book training, particularly acquisition training, can be conducted in a group, many members need additional individual therapy, which may be conducted alongside group therapy. Patients who require a great amount of drill work and reinforcement should not be placed in groups with those who learn more quickly and will soon advance to completing errands successfully. In these instances, it may become difficult to address both the needs of the advanced patient and the needs of average or slow-learning patients. Patients can be advanced to another group that addresses prospective memory and expects greater independence from the individual. In an advanced memory group, group work can be particularly useful, because people can schedule events with each other and be responsible to a peer rather than to the therapist only. As an example, a patient (Kevin) might include on his "to-do" list "Meet John outside Occupational Therapy to deliver letter from Mary" or "Meet John outside Physical Therapy to go to cafeteria." John's schedule would also include "Meet Kevin outside Physical Therapy to go to lunch," thus creating a checks-and-balances system. Clinicians, too, should model the use of an organizer by scheduling appointments, making "to-do" lists, and writing down reminders in their own organizers. As an example, whenever I schedule an appointment with a patient, I always make a point of saying, "Let me get my organizer and write it down, so I will be certain to remember." If I need to return to my office, I ask the patient to accompany me so that I can write the appointment in my organizer. When conducting a memory group, I always bring my organizer to the group and make entries in the group's presence.

Problem Solving and Executive Skills Training

Although problem solving, planning, self-awareness, self-monitoring, and other executive functions are addressed in the late stages of cognitive recovery, most often in post-acute rehabilitation settings, groups designed to focus on these skills are discussed in Chapter 16. Regardless of whether the treatment setting is in the community or part of a medical facility, at this stage of recovery, treatment should have a focus on community re-entry, which includes home, school, and work.

REIMBURSEMENT ISSUES

In the current competitive market, health care organizations and single providers are greatly challenged to bill for their services in a way that is reimbursable. Because services can be coded in a variety of ways (e.g., speech and language therapy, cognitive rehabilitation, group treatment), billing for treatment is not as straightforward as one might think. This is particularly true in the field of TBI rehabilitation because of the wide range of services that can be provided and because of the range of third-party payers. Private insurance includes not only medical but also automobile, homeowner's, and business liability; Medicare and Medicaid; vocational rehabilitation; school contracts; workers' compensation; and legal settlements.

Unlike the older population of people who have had a stroke, the younger TBI population does not have Medicare as a primary funding source for intensive rehabilitation. After a 2-year period of disability, some people may become eligible for Medicare services, but at that point, Medicare typically does not provide coverage for rehabilitation services to address long-standing problems. I make this point because some clients become eligible for Medicare while

still in need of treatment. At that point, either they or their representatives expect clinicians to deliver a new round of intensive therapy under the assumption that Medicare reimburses for the services. In my practice experience, unless a new condition or a change in condition arises that warrants rehabilitation, Medicare is not a reimbursement source for ongoing therapy.

State-funded and federally funded vocational rehabilitation programs often provide funding for people who have a vocational outlook. Sometimes, these programs even provide for people who do not have vocational potential but who, by having increased independence, allow a caregiver to return to work. Because these are state-managed programs, the criteria for services vary from state to state. Typically, however, service providers are expected to direct treatment toward goals related to a vocational outcome. Many organizations are able to negotiate contracts with vocational rehabilitation programs that may be based on a per diem rate and include a range of services. To reduce costs, private insurance companies may also negotiate per diem rates with facilities that provide a range of treatment options or several hours of therapy per day. Providing group therapy as a large part of the treatment day can make negotiated per diem rates an economic advantage for providers as well as payers.

Financial arrangements with third-party payers, such as those described above, drive many billing practices. Although an organization may establish pricing, clinicians often decide how a service is coded or billed. A great burden is thereby placed on clinicians to police their own billing practices. For example, patient John Doe has medical benefits through a health maintenance organization (HMO). The plan includes a certain number of visits to a speech-language pathologist. A visit is not defined in terms of length of session or method of delivery (i.e., group or individual). The reimbursement for the visit is half of what the fee structure of the organization has established for the service at an hourly rate. For example, the organization routinely charges $100 for an hour of individual therapy and $65 for an hour of group therapy, but the HMO pays $50 for a "visit." In this scenario, there is little incentive for the clinician to provide more than 30 minutes of individual or group therapy, although longer sessions may be indicated. Although providing group treatment would result in less "financial loss" to the provider, it may not be appropriate; but should it be made available? Thus, the payment source often dictates the service clinicians provide. This example demonstrates why many rehabilitation programs use a group treatment model for cost effectiveness. If the pricing structures of the organizations or payers vary greatly, one might have to distinguish between treating people in a group (and billing individually or at a group rate) and group therapy. The array of payment sources for TBI rehabilitation makes the financial aspects as challenging as the treatment itself. Although many different types and amounts of payment may be accepted, it is unethical and illegal to charge different providers different rates, especially if the provider participates in the Medicare program. Billing for cotreatment and treatment conducted in a community setting is discussed in Chapter 16.

REFERENCES

1. Gillis RJ, Pierce JN. Mechanisms of Traumatic Brain Injury and the Pathophysiologic Consequences. In RJ Gillis (ed), Traumatic Brain Injury Rehabilitation for Speech-Language Pathologists. Boston: Butterworth–Heinemann, 1996;38–57.
2. Gennarelli TA. Cerebral Concussion and Diffuse Brain Injuries. In PR Cooper (ed), Head Injury (3rd ed). Baltimore: Williams & Wilkins, 1993;137–158.
3. Hartley LL, Levin HS. Linguistic deficits after closed head injury: a current appraisal. Aphasiology 1990;4:353–370.
4. Hagen C, Malkmus D, Durham P. Levels of Cognitive Functioning. In Rehabilitation of the Head Injured Adult: Comprehensive Physical Management. Downey, CA: Professional Staff Association of Rancho Los Amigos Hospital, 1979.
5. Hagen C. Language Disorders in Head Trauma. In AL Holland (ed), Language Disorders in Adults: Recent Advances. San Diego: College Hill Press, 1984;245–281.
6. Adamovich BB, Henderson JA, Auerbach S. Cognitive Rehabilitation of Closed Head Injured Patients: A Dynamic Approach. San Diego: College Hill Press, 1985.
7. Kennedy MR, DeRuyter F. Cognitive and Language Bases for Communication Disorders. In DR Beukelman, KM Yorkston (eds), Communicative Disorders following Traumatic Brain Injury: Management of Cognitive, Language, and Motor Impairments. Austin, TX: Pro-Ed, 1991;123–190.
8. Szekeres SF, Ylvisaker M, Cohen SB. A Framework for Cognitive Rehabilitation Therapy. In M Ylvisaker, EM Gobble (eds), Community Re-entry for Head Injured Adults. Boston: College Hill Press, 1987;87–136.
9. Prigatano G, Fordyce DJ, Zeiner HK, et al. Neuropsychological Rehabilitation after Brain Injury. Baltimore: Johns Hopkins University Press, 1986.
10. Gronwall D, Wrightson P. Delayed recovery of intellectual function after minor head injury. Lancet 1974;2:605–609.
11. von Zomeren AH, Brouwer WH, Deelman BG. Attentional Deficits: The Riddles of Selectivity, Speed, and Alertness. In DN Brooks (ed), Closed Head Injury: Psychological, Social, and Family Consequences. Oxford: Oxford University Press, 1984;74–107.
12. Brooks DN. Cognitive Deficits. In M Rosenthal, ER Griffith, MR Bond, JD Miller (eds), Rehabilitation of the Adult and Child with Traumatic Brain Injury (2nd ed). Philadelphia: FA Davis, 1990;163–178.
13. Levin HS. Memory deficit after closed-head injury. J Clin Exp Neuropsychol 1989;12:129–153.
14. Stuss DT, Mateer CA, Sohlberg MM. Innovative Approaches to Frontal Lobe Deficits. In MAJ Finlayson, SH Garner (eds), Brain Injury Rehabilitation: Clinical Considerations. Baltimore: Williams & Wilkins, 1994;212–237.
15. Weddell R, Oddy M, Jenkins D. Social adjustment after rehabilitation: a two year follow-up of patients with severe head injury. Psychol Med 1980;10:257–263.
16. Livingston MG, Brooks DN, Bond MR. Patient outcome in the year following severe head injury and relatives' psychiatric and social functioning. J Neurol Neurosurg Psychiatry 1985;48:876–881.
17. Newton A, Johnson DA. Social adjustment and interaction after severe head injury. Br J Clin Psychol 1985;24:225–234.
18. Brooks DN (ed). Closed Head Injury: Psychological, Social, and Family Consequences. Oxford: Oxford University Press, 1984.
19. Ylvisaker M (ed). Head Injury Rehabilitation: Children and Adolescents. San Diego: College Hill Press, 1985.
20. Sohlberg MM, Mateer CA. Introduction to Cognitive Rehabilitation: Theory and Practice. New York: Guilford Press, 1989.
21. Beukelman DR, Yorkston KM (eds). Communicative Disorders following Traumatic Brain Injury: Management of Cognitive, Language and Motor Impairments. Austin, TX: Pro-Ed, 1991.
22. Long CJ, Ross LK (eds). Handbook of Head Trauma: Acute Care to Recovery. New York: Plenum, 1992;165–190.
23. Finlayson MAJ, Garner SH (eds). Brain Injury Rehabilitation: Clinical Considerations. Baltimore: Williams & Wilkins, 1994.
24. Hartley LL. Cognitive-Communicative Abilities following Brain Injury: A Functional Approach. San Diego: Singular Publishing, 1995.
25. Ben-Yishay Y. Working Approaches to Remediation of Cognitive Deficits in Brain Damaged Persons. New York: New York University Medical Center, 1980.
26. Ben-Yishay Y, Rattok J, Lakin P, et al. Neuropsychologic rehabilitation: quest for a holistic approach. Semin Neurol 1985;5:252–259.
27. Deaton AN. Group Interventions for Cognitive Rehabilitation: Increasing the Challenges. In JS Kreutzer, PH Wehman (eds), Cognitive Rehabilitation for People with Traumatic Brain Injury: A Functional Approach. Baltimore: Paul H. Brooks, 1991;191–200.
28. Ellis DW, Rader MA. Structured Sensory Stimulation. In CF Bontke (ed), Physical Medicine and Rehabilitation: State of the Art Reviews, vol 4. Philadelphia: Hanley and Belfus, 1990;465–477.
29. Wood RL. Critical analysis of the concept of sensory stimulation for patients in vegetative states. Brain Injury 1991;5:401–409.
30. Ansell BJ, Keenan JE. The Western Neuro Sensory Stimulation Profile: a tool for assessing slow to recover head injured patients. Arch Phys Med Rehabil 1989;70:104–108.
31. Radar MA, Ellis DW. The Sensory Stimulation Assessment Measure (SSAM): a tool for early evaluation of severely brain-injured patients. Brain Injury 1994;8:309–321.
32. Levin HS, O'Donnell VM, Grossman RG. The Galveston Orientation and Amnesia Test: a practical scale to assess cognition after head injury. J Nerv Ment Dis 1979;167:675–684.
33. Corrigan JD, Arnett JA, Houck LJ, Jackson RD. Reality orientation for brain injured patients: group treatment and monitoring of recovery. Arch Phys Med Rehabil 1985;66:626–630.
34. Sohlberg MM, Mateer CA. Effectiveness of an attention-training program. J Clin Exp Neuropsychol 1987;9:117–130.
35. Schacter DL, Crovitz HF. Memory function after closed head injury: a review of the quantitative research. Cortex 1977;13:150–176.
36. Gianutsos R, Gianutsos J. Rehabilitating the verbal recall of brain-injured patients by mnemonic training: an experimental demonstration using single-case methodology. J Clin Neuropsychol 1979;2:117–135.
37. Haarbauer-Krupa J, Moser L, Smith G, et al. Cognitive Rehabilitation Therapy: Middle Stages of Recovery. In M Ylvisaker (ed), Head Injury Rehabilitation: Children and Adolescents. San Diego: College Hill Press, 1985;287–310.
38. Mateer CA, Sohlberg MM. A Paradigm Shift in Memory Rehabilitation. In HA Whitaker (ed), Neuropsychological Studies of Non-focal Brain Damage: Dementia and Trauma. London: Springer-Verlag, 1988;202–225.
39. Sohlberg MM, Mateer CA. Training use of compensatory memory books: a three-stage behavioral approach. J Clin Exp Neuropsychol 1989;11:871–891.

CHAPTER SIXTEEN

Cotreatment and Community-Oriented Group Treatment for Traumatic Brain Injury

Rita J. Gillis

PHILOSOPHY OF COMMUNITY RE-ENTRY

Community re-entry has been used in traumatic brain injury (TBI) rehabilitation to mean both a goal of rehabilitation and a type of rehabilitation program. In general, there are no specific criteria for a community re-entry program. Programs may be located in freestanding rehabilitation centers, clinics, renovated homes, churches, schools, shopping centers, or office buildings. Programs may be residential or outpatient. They may include a supported work setting or not, but all have the primary focus of helping individuals develop the skills they need to function as community members and to identify and use the resources in their communities. Community re-entry programs should not only design treatment to simulate community activities, they should also conduct therapy in the community. As such, these programs must be located near resources such as a mall, library, grocery store, restaurant, bank, post office, and medical center and have access to transportation.

There are many reasons to work with individuals in a group format in a community re-entry program. First, groups in and of themselves are a type of small community; they provide socialization and require interdependence and cooperation. Second, generalization is a goal of therapy with all client populations, but it is particularly challenging for those with TBI because of difficulty in learning and transfer of learning. Target behaviors do not spontaneously carry over into natural contexts. Treatment that occurs in small isolated rooms does not provide sufficient exemplars or enough variety of experience for individuals to practice newly learned skills. Groups provide experience with different peers, therapists, and settings. Groups should be conducted in the community, or in a more natural setting, so that members can observe how behaviors are reinforced by or within the community. This can provide both patients and clinicians with insight. Skills that are not reinforced naturally in the environment by producing desired results are not maintained.

TYPES OF GROUPS FOR THE COMMUNITY RE-ENTRY SETTING

In a community re-entry setting, any number of groups can be conducted, either solely by speech-language pathologists or with therapists from other disciplines. Both types of groups are discussed. The types of groups that are managed solely by speech-language pathologists depend, in part, on the setting and the number of other disciplines involved. A small program may not employ a vocational specialist, yet may enroll a number of patients who are seeking employment. The speech-language pathologist can conduct a job communication group, for example, and may accompany patients into the community to job interviews, job fairs, or some similar activity. In a different setting with more staff, the same type of group might be co-facilitated by a speech-language pathologist and vocational specialist or occupational therapist. The types of groups discussed below can be directed only by a speech-language

pathologist but may include another discipline. For the most part, TBI rehabilitation is a team job that requires much cooperation and flexibility from the therapists. Clinicians who are territorial and uncomfortable in working with other therapists may find that teamwork is not an area of specialization for them. Most groups that exceed four members, and sometimes fewer, should have more than one therapist involved simply to observe behaviors and document performance.

Groups that address problem solving, reasoning, executive functions, and conversational and social skills are thought of as targeting multiple skills. The "higher-level cognitive skills" are multiprocess by definition. As such, it is difficult to single out separate processes, which may not even be desirable from a "functional" perspective [1]. The goal of functionality, however, should not encourage clinicians to develop groups that target a range of behaviors too vast to monitor carefully. At the community re-entry stage, it is particularly easy for clinicians to lose focus in an array of community-oriented activities and outings. Even if multiprocess or integrated skills could be broken down into their components, it would be impossible to develop different groups to address each of them. It is not impossible, however, to define specific goals for each group that can be addressed in stages and then to set only a few goals for each group member to accomplish at each stage. For example, in a pragmatics group, the first stage might focus only on the identification of pragmatic behaviors or the purposes of communication, instead of ten separate goals to address turn-taking, use of social rituals, maintaining topic, monitoring proximity, varying facial expression, and so on. It simply becomes difficult to monitor performance when groups try to accomplish too many goals simultaneously. Similarly, when groups go into the community, this provides an opportunity to observe many skills, but each therapist should define a limited set of behaviors to observe, cue, and review on return. Additionally, because people in community re-entry settings are often quite diverse in their range of skills, and there may not be enough like individuals to group by level, clinicians often must decide whether to advance activities when part of the group is ready and another is not. These are manageable problems in conducting group therapy, but they should be considered in advance. One method I have used to address differences in skill level within a group is to ask a patient with advanced skills to work with another patient whose skills are not as good. Using this method, I review the activities to use with both patients and obtain agreement between them about the way the practice sessions will occur. Then, I let them schedule the sessions based on a recommended frequency. This works particularly well in community re-entry programs, where patients often have down time between therapy sessions. Cooperative work also reinforces an interdependence model of community living.

Planning and Problem-Solving Groups

Problem-solving and executive skills are commonly listed as areas of impairment after a TBI, as noted in Chapter 15.

Most programs at the community re-entry level should have a problem-solving or similar group. It is difficult to separate planning from solving a problem because a variety of planning situations can be conceptualized as problems (e.g., a spouse's fiftieth birthday). Conversely, many problems require planning to solve.

The aim of treatment for problem-solving deficits is to impose a structure on a process that is often automatic or requires little deliberation for uninjured people. The ability to assess a situation quickly and have an immediate awareness of possible solutions is often diminished after a TBI. The ability to develop a plan or to recognize that a plan is needed also is often diminished. Before introducing problems to a group, it is necessary to teach members a problem-solving model or a step approach to solving problems. Problem-solving guides are taught to individuals with TBI because normal automaticity and awareness often are not available to them; they must learn *how* to conceptualize or think about particular situations so that goals can be accomplished. We all improve our problem-solving abilities because of feedback, either through our own trial and error or that of others, or from constructive criticism. Problem-solving groups offer opportunities for all three types of feedback.

Several models or guides for problem solving have been presented [2,3]. Models usually vary in terms of the number of steps taught, but five essential steps are common to most models. First, the problem has to be identified or recognized as it occurs. Second, the characteristics of the problem need to be defined. This aspect might include questioning, such as "How much of a problem is it? Is it a safety issue or an inconvenience? Does it need a solution?" and so on. This step concerns how one conceptualizes the problem, which affects how it will be solved. The third step is the generation and exploration of possible solutions or approaches to the problem. This includes evaluating the merit of each solution so that the best one can be implemented. It may include developing a plan, if multiple steps are required to implement the solutions. The fourth step is to implement the solution or plan. The final step in all models is to evaluate the effectiveness of the solution. In the first session of a problem-solving group, clinicians must provide the members with a guide to use. Part of the initial session should be devoted to a discussion of problem solving and trying to elicit steps from the group members themselves. Using steps that can be cued by an acronym is helpful. I have used the approach described by Bransford and Stein [4], which is cued by the acronym IDEAL:

- Identifying the problem
- Defining the problem
- Exploring alternative approaches
- Acting on the plan
- Looking at the effects

Table 16-1 presents an example of a problem-solving group that first teaches a problem-solving model and advances to planning a complicated activity to solve a problem. This type of group could be co-facilitated by an occupational therapist or another speech-language pathologist.

TABLE 16-1.
Example of a Planning and Problem-Solving Group

Staff-to-patient ratio: 1:4
Frequency: 4–5 times weekly
Group size: 4–6
Goals for group
- List the steps to problem-solving model.
- Identify each step as it is used in a problem situation.
- Apply the step procedure to sample problems.
- Solve problems in the rehabilitation setting using the model.
- Solve problems in the community using the model.

Suggestions for individual goals: For each group goal that must be accomplished in sequence, individual goals may vary in terms of percentages. Individuals who are unable to meet the first and second goals at 90–100% should be discharged or treated individually.

Sample problem activities

Play videotapes (of television shows or videos created by therapists) of problem situations where each step can be identified. Replay the recording until each step has been recognized.

Present hypothetical problems to the group, and ask them to apply the model. An example is "Mary and Steve were having a pool party. Two hours before the party Mary went outside to check the cleanliness of the pool. She walked across the deck and tripped on a board that had come loose and split."

Create problems in the group setting for members to solve. For example, unplug the television set or the videotape player and give one of the members a tape to play. Remove some of the chairs before the group arrives. Schedule two groups to meet in the same room.

Give the group a large problem to solve that requires planning and group cooperation. For example, tell the group that you want to move the furniture from one room into another with their help. Choose a smaller room, in which it will be difficult to fit the furniture but not so obvious that one could be certain without measuring.

Create a reason for the group to raise money and then have the group plan a fundraising event or activity, such as a bake sale, rummage sale, or pancake breakfast. Ensure that the facility has adequate resources to accomplish the event (e.g., a kitchen, supplies, staff or visitors to participate).

Foil a group outing, such as eating at a restaurant, by planning it at a place that is closed or not accessible. Therapists accompany the group but do not solve the problem.

The types of problem-solving and reasoning activities that speech-language pathologists are probably most familiar with are those that require verbalization of appropriate responses or possible solutions. An example of this type of problem is "What would you do if your neighbor's dog barked all night and kept you awake?" Many commercially available workbooks are filled with examples of this type, which may be one reason they commonly are used. Although this type of hypothetical problem solving using a question-and-answer format may have some benefit, unless it is modified it probably does little to help individuals learn a process or learn to self-evaluate their solutions. Too often when these types of problems are presented, clinicians rely on their own feedback exclusively for analyzing the effectiveness and appropriateness of the solutions, even in a group format. These types of problems can be used successfully in a group setting when other members of the group evaluate the appropriateness or effectiveness of the solutions and a printed scale or guide is used. This guide should give patients more definitive

TABLE 16-2.
Scales to Evaluate Solutions to Problems

Scale A

1	Very effective	Solves the problem with minimal consequences
2	Effective	Solves the problem, but with possible undesirable consequences
3	Ineffective	Does not solve the problem

Scale B

1	Very effective	Solves the problem with minimal consequences
2	Very effective	Solves the problem, but with possible severe consequences
3	Minimally effective	Partially or temporarily solves the problem, but with no consequences or repercussions
4	Ineffective	Does not solve the problem
5	Ineffective	Does not solve the problem and creates negative consequences

Note: Points on the scales are nominal and have no real ranking value.

feedback than something like, "Well, no, that's really not a good solution. Can you think of another one?" Using scales like those presented in Table 16-2 gives structure to a process that is similar to using a problem-solving guide such as IDEAL.

If the group is more advanced in both analytic abilities and flexibility, a more detailed scale (e.g., scale B in Table 16-2) could be used to increase discussion and analysis of problems and solutions. A scale should not have so many points that it becomes difficult to make distinctions, however, or it will be more confusing than helpful.

Using a scale can assist individuals in developing the evaluative aspects of problem solving. Sometimes individuals may know that a solution does not work but be unable to determine why it does not address the problem, which then makes it difficult to generate a better solution. A scale should be explained before being used in any group, and members should generate examples to represent each point on the scale. The majority of members should be able to represent each point on the scale with one example before attempting to rate the hypothetical problem situations. Once this has been accomplished, the scale can be used.

Because their thought is disorganized, the TBI patient's verbal expression is often disorganized and lacks fluency. Many activities designed to improve reasoning skills, such as analogies and convergent and divergent thinking tasks, are often thought of as verbal reasoning tasks (unless materials are graphic or nonverbal, as many are). Numerous paper-and-pencil activities and computer programs are used to address reasoning, but many of these activities are not functional. Although problems in verbal reasoning may underlie poor verbal expression, little if any evidence exists to indicate that targeting reasoning with either expressive or nonexpressive activities improves verbal expression. For example, although simple convergent thinking activities (e.g., what do a doughnut, tire, and lifesaver have in common?) may be used in a group to address verbal reasoning and expression, it is highly suspect that these exercises will improve the ability to express ideas, opinions, and feelings. At this stage of

rehabilitation, individuals need practice in expressing themselves.

Goals that specifically target verbal expression can be readily addressed in a group and are perhaps most appropriately addressed in groups. Again, the benefit of using a group format rather than individual therapy is the opportunity to practice in a social context, to learn from others through modeling, and to receive feedback from multiple sources. Table 16-3 is an example of a type of group that can be used to focus on verbal expression. Although similar activities can be used in groups that focus more on conversational discourse and pragmatics, clinicians may find that some individuals need more opportunity than just one type of group to practice verbal expression.

The form presented in Figure 16-1 is one way to help individuals understand the importance of the listener in determining whether information has been conveyed clearly. It is an example only and can be adapted to use with many of the activities in Table 16-3. Although verbal discussion is beneficial and can be well received by some, the importance of providing concrete feedback cannot be stressed enough. All groups at this stage need to help individuals develop evaluative skills, which are so important to self-reflection and self-monitoring.

Communication Groups

Communication group means any type of group whose goal is improved communication for socialization. These groups may go by many names, such as *conversational skills group, pragmatics group, group communication, social skills group,* and so on. Although it is recognized that communication, conversation, pragmatics, and social skills are not the same, the differences seem minor from an impairment perspective. The differences in terminology often reflect discipline differences rather than differences in group objectives. Communication groups are one of the few types of group intervention for TBI that have been researched and discussed by a variety of clinicians [5–8]. In part, this is because problems in social behavior are frequently reported as a major obstacle to positive reintegration after TBI. The skills to be addressed in communication groups include knowing the intent of communication and using a variety of communicative acts; being able to monitor the verbal and nonverbal behavior of oneself and others; knowing and being able to contribute to the topic of a communication exchange; and being able to understand (at some level) the perspective of speakers and listeners. These skills may be addressed through conversational discourse, debate, lectures, storytelling, role-play, and so on. Additionally, several communication groups may be held simultaneously in a facility that address different aspects. In my opinion, it is preferable to develop several different communication groups with specific functions or goals than to develop only one large group that attempts to meet the varied goals and needs of many individuals. Group structure, however, depends largely on the number of patients. Admittedly, it is difficult to organize several different communication groups or sub-

TABLE 16-3.
Example of a Verbal Expression Group

Staff-to-patient ratio: 1:6 if patients are highly similar; 1:4 if variable in skills
Group size: 4–6
Frequency: 2–5 times weekly
Goals for group
- Make distinctions between clear and concise statements and wordy or extraneous statements.
- State opinions and ideas concisely (i.e., without extraneous or excessive comments).
- Provide clear directions.
- Give personal information and express feelings or attitudes concisely.
- Use analogies to express opinions and ideas.
- Respond to situations with appropriate comments and emotional tone.

Suggestions for individual goals: Individual percentages or frequencies can be established for each goal for each member. These goals are not hierarchic, and many may be addressed simultaneously, but subgoals or short-term goals should be developed. For example, an individual who has difficulty relaying personal information concisely may be asked to state *no more than* five personal facts (in response to a question). Another individual who has difficulty thinking of and expressing personal information may be asked to state *at least* five personal facts.

Sample activities

Have members state the pros and cons of different situations relevant to members of the group (e.g., What are the advantages of using [or learning to use] the public transportation system?). First, discuss the meaning of pros and cons or advantages and disadvantages.

Have members state their opinions about events or procedures that occur in the rehabilitation setting and about news events from the community. The pros-and-cons dichotomy helps to keep opinions focused.

Describe personal events or situations, and ask members to describe an analogous situation either from their own experience or from that of someone they know.

Print hypothetical (but realistic) situations on cards that require a verbal response. Give each member a card to which a verbal response can be given. Other members are asked to judge the response (see Figure 16-1) based on how well they could guess the situation and to judge the appropriateness or effectiveness of the response in terms of emotional tone (e.g., too angry, not forceful enough, didn't convey being upset).

Examples of situations to print on cards:
- You are in your boss's office and have just been told that you're fired as of today.
- You are at a MacDonald's drive-through and have checked your order, which has fries, a hamburger, and a soda. You ordered a fish sandwich and a chocolate milkshake.
- Your friend is on the phone and says she can't bring you your wallet that you left at her house last night, even though she said she would bring it to you at 5 P.M. today. You need to go to the grocery store at 6 P.M., when your ride comes.
- Last week you ordered a shirt (size medium) from a mail-order catalog. It arrived yesterday but is too small. You are on the phone with the company now.

Have members give directions to their place of residence or some other known location in the community. Other members can judge whether they think they could get to the location based on the directions.

Have members tell how to perform a procedural task that has been written on a card. Give each member a card with a relevant task that he or she knows how to perform. Other members should be able to guess the task, but they also can be asked to judge the quality of the instructions.

Ask each member to relay some type of personal information to the group. Examples include these:
- What is your best feature or characteristic?
- What was your worst hospital experience?
- Who has influenced you the most and why?
- What did you like about high school, college, your job, etc.?
- What is something you do well?

Each member can have a different question, and members can generate questions to ask each other.

groups if your facility has only four patients who can be grouped successfully. When facilities have small numbers of similar patients, it is often more effective to have one or two groups that address different aspects of communication in different sessions. This is true for all groups, not just communication groups. For example, on Monday, Wednesday, and Friday a group might address turn-taking and pause time, and on Tuesday and Thursday the same group could address aspects of nonverbal communication, such as proximity, eye contact, and facial expressions.

Unlike some of the other cognitive skills that have been discussed, many scales evaluating the communication skills of people with TBI either have been, or can be, used in a group. No single scale has been evaluated thoroughly in this population. This is not surprising, in view of the relative newness of assessing pragmatics and social skills. Most scales are inventories of skills or simple rating systems. Table 16-4 lists some of the scales used in this population, with a brief description of the characteristics. The scales vary considerably in detail of the ratings used and range of communicative behaviors rated.

These scales can be used to provide clinicians with an initial impression of the pragmatic or communication abilities of the group members. However, most of the scales listed in Table 16-4 are too cumbersome for routine recording of target behaviors. As such, clinicians may choose to use portions of a scale or inventory that assess only the behaviors to be targeted during the group. If group members are to assess each other's behavior, or are to rate their own, clinicians may choose to develop a check-off system that can be easily interpreted and used. In the author's experience, documentation of group progress is more manageable when clinicians use the same forms for rating behaviors of group members. An example of a communication group designed to assist people in understanding and using a variety of communication intents is presented in Table 16-5. Figure 16-2 gives an example of a check-off system that could be used with the group members to identify different intents.

The communication activities presented in Table 16-5 focus on improving one aspect of communication. An entire group may be devoted to communication acts, or they may be addressed as a phase of training in a group that addresses a wider array of communication behaviors. How the group is structured is not of primary importance. It is of primary importance, however, that awareness training be conducted at length before people are expected to modify behaviors. The same example presented in Figure 16-2 can be followed to modify any number of behaviors, such as facial expressions, vocal intensity and tone, turn-taking, topic maintenance, understanding nonverbal cues, and so on. Communication groups offer many opportunities to address self-awareness, monitoring, self-regulation, initiation, and other "executive skills." These skill areas are often impaired, and their impairment is reflected in poor social interactions. It is important that a systematic approach be taken in communication training and that patients not be bombarded with feedback about all the inappropriate behaviors at one time.

Group member name *(i.e., the person responding to the situation)*:

Mark an X in the box to show how well you understood the situation.

☐   Knew exactly the situation and the person(s) involved.

Describe:

☐   Somewhat knew the situation but have some questions.

Describe or ask questions:

☐   Have no idea.

Was the member's tone appropriate or inappropriate? *(Circle the word)*

FIGURE 16-1.
Form to judge completeness of verbal expression. (Items in italics are descriptors for the readers. The instructions for using the form can be given orally to the members.)

COTREATMENT IN COMMUNITY RE-ENTRY PROGRAMS

Groups taken into the community should always be accompanied by more than one therapist and, depending on the focus of the group or of the activity, the therapists may be all speech-language pathologists or from several disciplines. There are many advantages to working with other therapists when conducting groups in the community. The safety and welfare of the patients is of utmost concern, and merely leaving the protective confines of a clinic setting increases the risks. Of course, clinicians should not take into the community individuals about whom they know very little in terms of behavior and skills. It is necessary to be able to anticipate the reactions of patients in public places to the extent possible, and this requires knowing the patients beyond a highly structured evaluation setting. Individuals with TBI can become quickly overwhelmed in unfamiliar situations, and clinicians should be prepared for the unexpected. In this area, two clinicians' heads are better than one. Additionally, a community activity requires multiple skills of concern to many of the treating therapists. Because it is often difficult to make the arrangements and obtain the necessary consent for community activities, it is useful for several clinicians to be involved in the activity. Firsthand observation and the opportunity to intervene outside the clinic provide much more useful information to therapists than do verbal reports. For example, the speech-language pathologist observes a communication exchange between a store clerk and a patient more critically than would a physical

therapist who was focusing primarily on mobility, but it is important to observe both skills.

Cost effectiveness is another reason to conduct activities in the community with a group of patients and more than one therapist. It is rarely cost effective to use a facility's transportation to send one patient into the community or to arrange for a taxi. Because of the planning and additional expense involved in going into the community (if the destination is not within walking distance), a group community activity is a better use of clinical resources and it is often more fun for the clients.

Speech-Language Pathology and Occupational Therapy

Because occupational therapists and speech-language pathologists often address the same types of skills (e.g., reading, calculations, following directions), time and money can be wasted with duplication of effort. Therapists frequently are territorial, and each discipline thinks its approach is best. Groups comanaged by occupational therapy and speech-language pathology, however, can provide some of the most functional activities for patients at this stage of rehabilitation, if they have a genuinely cooperative approach and groups are planned carefully. Table 16-6 presents an example of a group that can be managed by occupational therapy and speech-language pathology. Criteria for inclusion are given as an example for therapists who may not be familiar with cotreatment groups.

Detailed criteria for inclusion and a time frame for ending the group are recommended for groups of this

TABLE 16-4.
Scales for Rating Communication Skills

Scale	Rating/Scoring	Behaviors
Profile of Functional Impairment in Communication [9]	0–5 rating: 0 = normal, 1 = very mildly impaired, 2 = mildly impaired, 3 = moderately impaired, 4 = severely impaired, 5 = very severely impaired. 0–3 rating for the presence of specific behaviors: 0 = not at all, 1 = occasionally, 2 = often/almost always, 3 = always, and a "not noted" option	Ten communication rules and 84 specific behavior items related to these rules: lexical content, general participation, quantity, quality, internal relation, external relation, clarity of expression, social style, subject matter, aesthetics. Example: The specific behaviors used in rating the feature scale for lexical content were anomia, bizarre utterance, circumlocutions, dysfluency, echolalia, fragmentation, neologism, paraphasias, peculiar phrases, and sentence complexity.
Conversational Rating Scale [10]	1–9 rating, with anchors described at the 1-, 3-, 5-, 7-, and 9-point ratings. Eye gaze example: 1 = consistently no appropriate eye gaze with another person, 3 = severely restricted eye gaze, 5 = appropriate eye gaze 50% of the time, 7 = appropriate eye gaze 75% of the time, 9 = consistent use of appropriate eye gaze	Six behaviors: intelligibility, eye gaze, sentence formation, coherence of narrative, topic (maintenance), initiation of communication
Pragmatic Protocol [11]	Appropriate/inappropriate/no opportunity to observe	30 behaviors: Verbal/paralinguistic: intelligibility, vocal intensity, voice quality, prosody, fluency. Nonverbal: physical proximity, physical contacts, body posture, foot/leg movements and hand/arm movements, gestures, facial expression, eye gaze. Lexical selection/use: specificity/accuracy. Specifying relationships between words: cohesion. Stylistic variations: varying of communicative style. Speech acts: pair analysis, variety. Topic: selection, introduction, maintenance, change. Turn-taking: initiation, response, repair/revision, pause time, interruption/overlap, feedback to speaker, adjacency, contingency, quantity/concision
Conversational Skills Rating Scale (cited by Hartley [1] as useful with this population, but no research data are reported on its use)	1–5 rating: 1 = inadequate, 2 = somewhat inadequate, 3 = adequate, 4 = good, 5 = excellent. Additional rating of overall conversational performance with 1–5 rating on 5 parameters: 1 = poor conversationalist, 5 = excellent conversationalist; 1 = socially unskilled, 5 = socially skilled; 1 = incompetent interactant, 5 = competent interactant; 1 = inappropriate interactant, 5 = appropriate interactant; 1 = ineffective interactant, 5 = effective interactant	Twenty-five behaviors: speaking rate, speaking fluency, vocal confidence, articulation, vocal variety, volume, posture, lean toward partner, shaking or nervous twitches, unmotivated movements or fidgeting, use of eye contact, facial expressiveness, nodding of head in response to partner's statements, use of gestures to emphasize what was being said, smiling and/or laughing, use of humor and/or stories, asking questions, encouragements or agreements, speaking about partner or partner's interests, speaking about self, expression of personal opinions, initiation of new topics, maintenance of topics and follow-up comments, interruption of partner's speaking turns, use of time speaking relative to partner
Communication Performance Scale [7]	1–5 rating with end-points defined for each behavior. Example: variety of language uses, 1 = limited use of language, stereotypical language; 5 = uses language to express feelings, share information, social interaction	Thirteen behaviors: intelligibility, prosody/rate, body posture, facial expression, lexical selection, syntax, cohesiveness, variety of language uses, topic, initiation of conversation, repair, interruption, listening

TABLE 16-5.
Example of a Communication Group

Staff-to-patient ratio: 1:4
Group size: 4–8
Frequency: 3–5 times weekly
Goals for group
- List a minimum of 15 communicative intents.
- Identify a variety of communicative intents when used.
- Use a variety of communicative intents during group activities.

Suggestions for individual goals: The number of communicative intents or a percentage can be specified for each member and upgraded on a weekly basis. Some members may not be able to generate a minimum number but may still be able to identify the use of a variety of intents by using a check-off system or form.

Types of communicative intents: Telling/giving information, asking/seeking information, directing, demanding, asserting, refusing, criticizing, teasing, joking, agreeing, threatening, complimenting, encouraging, etc.

Sample activities

Discuss the purposes of communication and what communication intentions are. Try to have members generate as many examples as possible before using a form.

Play recordings of television shows with interactions that clearly display different intentions and have members mark them on a form when identified. Review as a group. The *Dick Van Dyke Show*, the *Mary Tyler Moore Show*, and *Bewitched* are good examples and easily obtained.

Using materials from above, single out one intent (e.g., instances of demanding or complimenting) and review the tape to count the instances observed. Compare tallies and review again as a group.

Give each member a card with a specific communicative intent to convey. Other members guess what it is.

Give each member a card with a specific situation or instruction and have each respond to the group. The group guesses the intention. For example, a card could read "Mary has accused you of taking her pen when she went to the restroom" or "A man approaches you on the corner of X and Y and asks for directions to the clinic."

---

type that have a specific goal to accomplish (e.g., actually prepare a meal). If the group includes members who have little experience in meal preparation and buying groceries, several sessions may have to be devoted to estimating costs, or members may receive additional sessions outside the group. A variety of activities and materials can be used to accomplish the goal of estimating costs. Sales fliers from local groceries can be reviewed to learn the costs of various foods. A mini-grocery store can be developed, with priced items. Plastic foods can be substituted for perishable items, and all materials can be stored in boxes, if space is an issue. Several lists of foods with a range of prices can be made up in advance, and clients can use the lists to determine costs. Any combination of activities can be used until all group members are able to generate a shopping list and budget the amount of money needed within an established range (e.g., $5).

One or more sessions should be devoted to reading recipes and understanding the complexity and amount of time required to prepare various items. After this, members can generate various menus, which can be judged for ease and nutritional value. These can be written on a board, where they can be compared and discussed. Additional time may have to be devoted to discussing balanced meals

before a menu is chosen. Time estimation and planning the use of the stove, oven, and limited utensils are variables to discuss when choosing menus for the final meal. Depending on what needs to be purchased, all or only some of the members may go to the grocery store. The length of time the group lasts is determined by the number of members, but sufficient time should be allotted for each member to prepare a meal, because that is the primary goal.

When planning a group of this nature, therapists must be organized. For example, recipe books may have to be brought from home. If the facility does not have a van, transportation must be arranged. This type of group requires more resources (both time and money) than do some other groups, but it can be very beneficial. It is an essential exercise for people who have the potential to live with greater independence but who may not have the necessary skills.

Job or Vocational Communication Groups

In the community re-entry setting, many people want to find employment or return to a job. Because of the relatively young age of the population, some have little experience in looking for jobs. Problems in communication and social skills may interfere with obtaining and keeping employment. Many rehabilitation settings have a vocational specialist with whom the speech-language pathologist can work on job-related communication skills. Many do not, however, and the group example presented in Table 16-7 can be carried out alone, with another speech-language pathologist, or with an occupational therapist. Although job-related communication activities are easily presented in another type of communication group, not all members in another group may have the shared goal of employment. For those who do, a specific vocational group may be indicated and can provide a greater focus on communication skills important to employment.

Once a week, or every 2 weeks, members of the vocational communication group should go into the community to practice some of the skills being addressed. Job fairs provide an opportunity for all members to go to the same place, but these are not always available. With some planning, however, other types of opportunities can be arranged. For example, the group could go to a large employer, such as a hospital or school, and meet with the human resources director or an administrator. They could inquire about the types of jobs available, the minimal requirements, the desired requirements, how many people with disabilities are employed, and so on. These created opportunities are not necessarily meant to lead to employment but to provide members with exposure to and practice with real employers.

Other Types of Co-facilitated Groups

Because communication is a skill that transcends disciplines, speech-language pathologists can work with almost any other type of therapist. It is not necessary that an entire group be dedicated to a codiscipline approach to treat with another therapist. Often the speech-language pathologist

Name:	Date:
Communicative Intention	√ *Observed/number of times observed*
Accusing/blaming	
Agreeing	
Arguing	
Asking for information	
Asserting	
Begging/pleading	
Bragging/boasting	
Clarifying	
Comforting	
Complaining/whining	
Complimenting	
Criticizing	
Defending	
Demanding	
Directing	
Disagreeing	
Encouraging	
Giving information	
Joking/teasing/being sarcastic	
Promising	
Refusing	
Threatening	
Warning	

FIGURE 16-2.
Form to use for identifying communicative intentions.

can join another group for one session a week or every other week to observe patients in different situations and to provide feedback. For example, a physical therapy group can be conducted with an activity that requires giving and following directions, monitoring verbal output and appropriateness of responses, taking turns, initiating, and so on. It is not necessary that the speech-language pathologist develop a new goal for each member in the physical therapy group. Instead, one could choose a goal

that is being addressed in another type of group. If a patient in the physical therapy group is not one whom the speech-language pathologist treats in another group, that is fine, as long as that member is not accidentally billed.

Although many facilities, particularly transitional residential facilities, take patients on recreational outings (e.g., to a movie), in my experience, these are difficult for the speech-language pathologist to justify as a co-facilitator. The reasoning is that the recreational activity itself

TABLE 16-6.
Example of a Meal-Planning Group

Staff-to-patient ratio: 1:3 (occupational therapist, speech-language pathologist, and an assistant if more than six patients)
Group size: 6–8
Frequency: Daily
Duration: 8–10 weeks
Facility requirements: Stocked kitchen that is available at least once a week, funds to make food purchases
Criteria for inclusion
- Desires and has the potential to live semi-independently or independently
- Needs to prepare meals for himself or herself
- Can read simple words
- Can recognize numbers
- Can tell time
- Can follow verbal commands
- Knows the value of money
- Has the physical skills to use kitchen utensils and equipment (may be adaptive)
- Can communicate using simple phrases (may be augmentative or alternative)

Goals for the group
- Plan costs associated with preparing a well-balanced meal
- Follow directions to simple 5- to 8-step recipes
- Plan or sequence steps to preparing a meal
- Use safe kitchen practices when preparing a meal
- Estimate and monitor time
- Work with a group to complete multiple tasks
- Prepare a well-balanced meal with minimal assistance

Sample weekly objectives
Estimate costs associated with food items
Read directions from recipes
Generate* lists for items to purchase and tasks to complete
Generate* well-balanced menus
Estimate cooking times and schedule multiple tasks
Variables to consider and plan for: The maximum amount of time that is available to prepare and eat the meal, dividing meal preparation tasks among members before starting, amount of money available for food and drinks, transportation to the grocery store, spatial arrangement to accommodate all members. (Therapists must account for these variables to prevent disaster, but group members should be guided to consider these issues themselves when planning.)

*Should include writing down.

TABLE 16-7.
Example of Vocational Communication Group

Staff-to-patient ratio: 1:4
Group size: 4–8
Frequency: 3–5 times weekly
Goals for group
- Obtain and provide information over the phone regarding employment opportunities
- Ask pertinent questions and answer questions effectively during job interviews
- Understand job requirements and be able to discuss qualifications for various jobs
- Identify appropriate and inappropriate types of communication to use with supervisors and coworkers
- Use different types of communication appropriate to workers' positions

Suggestions for individual goals: Individual percentages can be established for each goal for each member. These goals are not hierarchic, and many may be addressed simultaneously, but subgoals or short-term goals should be developed. For example, individuals must identify questions to ask over the phone before making contacts.
Sample activities
Review a variety of job advertisements, and have members generate questions they would ask over the phone to learn more about positions. Have members rehearse with each other on the phone using the list.
Provide examples of appropriate and inappropriate comments to make to a supervisor, and have members decide if they are or are not appropriate and give reasons why. Repeat with examples of comments to coworkers of different sexes.
Have members provide examples of appropriate and inappropriate comments to make to a supervisor or topics to discuss with a supervisor or coworkers. Do the same with appropriate and inappropriate nonverbal behaviors.
Play videotapes of on-the-job communication interactions between supervisors and employees and between coworkers. Have members identify appropriate and inappropriate comments and behaviors.
Discuss the consequences of being "inappropriate" on the job.
Role-play interview situations. Provide members with specific scenarios. Have other members rate the effectiveness of the interviewer and interviewee.

should be the focus of the outing, and it is often difficult to devote enough time to communication goals to justify the use of the speech-language pathologist's skills. The speech-language pathologist, however, can be involved in groups designed to plan recreational outings with a recreational or leisure therapist. If recreational activities are routinely planned in the facility, a group might be formed specifically to address the planning aspects. This type of group could be developed in several ways. A planning and problem-solving group might already exist, and planning recreational activities could be one of the problems the group must solve. Alternately, if there is enough demand and resources, an entire group might be formed for the specific purpose of planning weekly recreational events. The goals would vary for the individuals in the group and would require a good deal of forethought by the clinicians to guide the assignment of duties to each patient based on need. The group might be labeled a leisure planning group or some variant.

This type of group can target the many cognitive-communicative skills that must be used to plan a leisure activity. These include reading, writing, verbal expression, organization, auditory comprehension, and initiation, to list a few. For the speech-language pathologist, this type of group would supplement other therapy sessions, but it might be a primary group for the leisure or recreation therapist. For example, a person who is working on listening and writing down information might be given the assignment of phoning theaters and obtaining a list of movies playing. Another person could be given the task of finding out the preferences of the group members and categorizing the responses (e.g., three people want to watch a comedy, two people want an action-adventure, one person wants a romantic movie). The assigned tasks for groups of this type do not necessarily need to be conducted during the group. Individual therapy sessions that target the specific needs of a person could use materials relevant to the group activity to meet the group's goals. For example, a person who is working on reading in individual therapy could be assigned the task of reading the movie schedules in the paper outside the group. This would be a more functional and relevant therapy material to use than a workbook selection. When the group reconvenes, the person has the necessary information for the group to make a decision.

DOCUMENTATION AND REIMBURSEMENT ISSUES

Documentation of group therapy can be greatly facilitated if standard observation tools are developed for each group and, in each group session, therapists narrow their scope to one or two behaviors for each patient. Several examples of forms and goals have been presented. When conducting a group with another therapist, such as the meal-planning group (see Table 16-6), each therapist can have his or her own goals for each patient. These goals may also be addressed in another therapy session with activities such as reading labels, recipes, and sales fliers. Activities can be divided between therapists based on their skill and level of comfort; then, each therapist has leadership responsibility for certain activities and sessions (e.g., reading recipes and generating menu options). Documentation in the patient's record either can be rotated based on the person who leads the session or divided by patient, depending on each patient's most apparent need (impairment).

Typically, the therapist who documents the session bills for the service. Because some facilities require therapists to bill for each session in which they participate, it may be necessary to divide the patients between clinicians for each session rather than rotating sessions. If providers charge by time, rather than a flat fee, each therapist can bill for half the session. The advantage of programs that are able to negotiate a per diem rate with payers is greater flexibility for therapists to cotreat and to go into the community.

Billing for group community outings can be handled in many ways and, again, depends on the organization and the funding sources. As an example, a physical therapist, a speech-language pathologist, and an occupational therapist accompany 10 patients to the community mall. Each person is expected to maneuver safely within the mall and stores using skills that have been targeted in the clinical setting, to ask for assistance in locating an item, and to make a purchase. These activities are monitored by each therapist: physical, speech-language, and occupational, respectively. The trip takes 3 hours. The three therapists might bill this activity in several ways. Each therapist might bill each patient for 1 hour of therapy at a group rate (assuming the group rate is lower). Because it is impossible for any of the therapists to spend enough time with any single patient, it would be difficult to justify billing at an individual rate for an hour. However, each therapist might bill each patient at an individual rate for a 15-minute session (or more, if additional time was spent with a particular patient). Alternatively, before the outing, each therapist would be assigned three to four patients based on their primary needs, such as communication or mobility. Then, each therapist could bill at a group rate for the patients for the full 3 hours. Clearly, billing decisions must be made *before* community outings, particularly if the latter billing method is chosen. If the speech-language pathologist had three patients for 3 hours as a group, there would certainly need to be a major emphasis on communication over mobility, and multiple communication opportunities would have to be provided.

It cannot be overstated that planning group therapy for individuals with TBI requires a great deal of effort and team cooperation. Unlike people with aphasia, language is not the greatest obstacle for many of these people. In fact, it is difficult to separate out a single obstacle. Therapists must be creative and sometimes go beyond the bounds of their academic training. As with any population, however, therapists should not exceed the limits of their knowledge. As always, it is necessary to establish goals, to monitor and document progress, and to discontinue therapy when progress cannot be observed.

REFERENCES

1. Hartley LL. Cognitive-Communicative Abilities following Brain Injury: A Functional Approach. San Diego: Singular Publishing, 1995.
2. Ben-Yishay Y. Working Approaches to Remediation of Cognitive Deficits in Brain Damaged Persons. New York: New York University Medical Center, 1980;129–174.
3. Ylvisaker M, et al. Topics in Cognitive Rehabilitation Therapy. In M Ylvisaker, EM Gobble (eds), Community Re-entry for Head Injured Adults. Boston: College Hill Press, 1987;137–220.
4. Bransford JD, Stein BS. The Ideal Problem Solver: A Guide for Improving Thinking, Learning, and Creativity. New York: Freeman, 1984.
5. Carlson HB, Buckwald MBW. Vocational communication group treatment in an outpatient head injury facility. Brain Inj 1993;7:183–187.
6. Boake C. Social Skills Training following Head Injury. In JS Kreutzer, PH Wehman (eds), Cognitive Rehabilitation for Persons with Traumatic Brain Injury: A Functional Approach. Baltimore: Paul H. Brookes, 1991;181–189.
7. Ehrlich J, Sipes A. Group treatment of communication skills for head trauma patients. Cogn Rehabil 1985;3:32–37.
8. Milton SB, Prutting CA, Binder GM. Appraisal of Communicative Competence in Head Injured Adults. In RH Brookshire (ed), Clinical Aphasiology Conference Proceedings. Minneapolis: BRK Publishers, 1984;114–123.
9. Linscott RJ, Knight RG, Godfrey HPD. The Profile of Functional Impairment in Communication (PFIC): a measure of communication impairment for clinical use. Brain Inj 1996;10:397–412.
10. Ehrlich J, Barry P. Rating communication behaviours in the head-injured adult. Brain Inj 1989;3:193–198.
11. Prutting CA, Kirchner DM. A clinical appraisal of the pragmatic aspects of language. J Speech Hear Disord 1987;52:105–119.

SECTION V

Motor Speech Disorders

CHAPTER SEVENTEEN

Group Therapy for Dysarthria

Mary Boyle,
Ann Marie Marchese,
and Christina V. Green

Our work setting is a 150-bed, not-for-profit inpatient rehabilitation facility that also provides outpatient treatment. The groups that we describe need not be restricted to this setting, but factors may be intrinsic to our setting that other clinicians might need to take into account to adapt these programs. We run two groups for inpatients who have dysarthria: a dysarthria group, which focuses on conversation, and an oral motor group for people who need to work on strengthening oral musculature. Both groups are ongoing, and patients move in and out of them as they move through their inpatient rehabilitation stay. Our outpatient dysarthria groups differ from the inpatient groups primarily in reimbursement issues and in their life span: They are established when a number of people can be appropriately grouped, they run for a specific number of weeks, and then they disband. All the groups described in this chapter are for adults.

INPATIENT DYSARTHRIA GROUPS

Philosophy of Program

This group was established because the speech-language pathologists felt a need to promote generalization of the techniques that patients were learning in individual treatment sessions. Although the clinicians included generalization activities in individual sessions, they felt limited by scheduling constraints, inability of family members or friends to attend sessions, and many other variables.

Because a group involves techniques for programming generalization [1], it seemed to be an efficient way to achieve our goal. It provides a variety of conversational partners, thus encouraging generalization across people. Some of these partners have hearing impairments, as do some group members' spouses, thus allowing the members the opportunity to practice compensatory strategies and environmental control techniques [2]. The group meets in a larger room than the individual sessions do, requiring the members to make the transition from close-proximity, one-to-one interactions with the clinician to larger distances between speakers. It also requires them to adapt to the dynamics of group conversation, which do not always allow for orderly turn-taking. These factors encourage generalization across settings and conditions while also encouraging the use of compensatory strategies and environmental control. The group provides less structured stimuli, responses, and reinforcement than the individual sessions, so it serves as a form of loose training and indistinguishable contingencies. Finally, the group provides natural maintaining contingencies to the extent that members are naturally reinforced for their successful communications in the group by the responses of the other members. Our previous experiences with group treatment suggested that people frequently respond better to peer feedback than to feedback, either positive or negative, from clinicians or spouses, and others have confirmed this observation [3].

The group, which meets once a week, is an adjunct to daily individual therapy for most participants. In some instances, if they progress to the point that generalization of compensatory strategies is their only remaining goal, the group might be the only speech-language therapy they receive. As the length of inpatient rehabilitation stay has decreased in the past few years, we have begun to consider the need for running the group more frequently (i.e., two or three times a week) so that people can attend more than one or two group sessions.

Entry Criteria

Candidates for this group are dysarthric inpatients whose conversational speech is at least moderately intelligible and whose performance during the assessment reveals the need to address goals of improving intelligibility in connected speech, promoting generalization of strategies to social interactions, improving motivation, or improving insights about their disability. If a patient has aphasia in addition to the dysarthria, the patient's primary clinician and the group coordinator confer to determine whether the patient's language abilities are good enough to allow the patient to benefit from the group experience.

Assessment

Patients are assessed individually on referral from the attending physician. The assessment includes the standard components, such as identifying information; medical, social, and educational history; reason for referral; and a hearing screening. The evaluation focuses on an oral peripheral examination of the structure and function of the oral articulators and observation and testing of respiration, phonation, resonance, articulation, and prosody in a variety of tasks. Instrumental assessment with the Iowa Oral Performance Instrument or the Visi-Pitch II, or both, is usually included. Other aspects of communication and swallowing are assessed as necessary. The results of the evaluation, including a diagnosis and prognosis, are explained to the individual and, if possible, to the family. Recommendations are made and goals are formulated with input from the patient and family.

If the person is somewhat intelligible on the conversational level during the assessment, a referral to the group is usually made immediately. If the person's conversational speech is unintelligible, individual treatment begins and group treatment is deferred until conversational speech is at least moderately intelligible.

Treatment Goals

Treatment goals are established individually for each patient during the assessment. The referring clinician indicates which goals the patient should be focusing on by checking them on the Dysarthria Group Referral Sheet/Report (Figure 17-1). Because many dysarthric people have had right cerebrovascular accidents that affected their pragmatic skills, we also include some pragmatic goals that we would like these individuals to work on in the group setting.

Patient's name: _____   Unit: _____

Speech-language pathologist: _____   Date: _____

Suggested Treatment Goals		Cueing (circle one)			Comments
_____ Diaphragmatic breathing	ind	min	mod	max	
_____ Coordination of respiration and phonation	ind	min	mod	max	
_____ Breath phrasing	ind	min	mod	max	
_____ Phonates consistently	ind	min	mod	max	
_____ Slower rate of speech	ind	min	mod	max	
_____ Pacing words or syllables	ind	min	mod	max	
_____ Exaggerated articulation	ind	min	mod	max	
_____ Opens mouth more widely when speaking	ind	min	mod	max	
_____ Increased loudness	ind	min	mod	max	
_____ Intonational variation	ind	min	mod	max	
_____ Managing secretions	ind	min	mod	max	

Other Goals

_____ Eye contact	ind	min	mod	max	
_____ Initiate one comment	ind	min	mod	max	
_____ Turn taking	ind	min	mod	max	
_____ Topic maintenance	ind	min	mod	max	

ind = patient initiates strategies without any reminders; mod = patient requires verbal cues about every other turn; min = patient requires fewer than 5 verbal cues during session; max = patient requires verbal cues every time she or he speaks.

FIGURE 17-1.

Burke Rehabilitation Hospital Speech-Language and Audiology Dysarthria Group Referral Sheet/Report. This form serves as both a referral sheet and documentation of the individual's performance. The referring clinician fills out the identifying information and checks off the appropriate goals. The clinician coordinating the group circles the level of cueing the patient required on each goal and makes relevant comments. The form is returned to the referring clinician, who includes the information in progress notes and the discharge summary. A new form is used for each patient in each group session.

When new patients are referred to the group, their primary clinician uses a handout (Figure 17-2) to explain the purpose of the group and to review the patient's goals. The patient is encouraged to share this handout with family members so that they are aware of the strategies we would like the patient to practice during conversation.

Documentation of Progress

The Dysarthria Group Referral Sheet/Report (see Figure 17-1) serves as the basis for documenting progress. The clinician who is coordinating the group indicates the level of cueing the patient required during the session and makes any comments relevant to the patient's performance; he or she then returns the form to the patient's primary clinician. The primary clinician uses the information to focus individual treatment for the patient and includes it in weekly progress notes and in the discharge summary.

Clinical Techniques

The size of the group varies depending on the number of dysarthric inpatients who are working on their speech at a conversational level. The groups have run with as few as

Your speech-language pathologist, _____, has recommended that you be a part of our Dysarthria Group. The purpose of this group is to work on making your speech as clear as possible by giving you extra practice in a conversational situation with other people who have similar speech problems.

    The group meets once a week on _____ at _____ in _____. The group coordinator is _____.

  You can be discharged from this group when you and your speech-language pathologist determine that your speech is understandable and you no longer need this extra practice.

  It is important for you to use the following strategies in this group (and whenever you talk) to make your speech as understandable as possible:

_____

_____

_____

_____

Speech-Language Pathologist, extension _____

FIGURE 17-2.

Burke Rehabilitation Hospital Speech-Language and Audiology Dysarthria Group handout for patients and families. This handout is given to new patients who are referred to the dysarthria group.

three members and as many as 12, but typically there are five to seven people in a group. The group is scheduled for an hour, but allowing for the time at the beginning and end for everyone to assemble and then to leave for their next appointment means that the group really meets for approximately 50 minutes.

The group is held in a large multipurpose room, with enough space to make a circle with wheelchairs. Because new people may join the group every week, the group begins with introductions. Participants state their names and where they live. This usually provokes some conversational exchanges from people who live, or used to live, in the same towns, or who know people in the town where another group member is from. After the introductions, the coordinator reviews the purpose of the group and explains that every member of the group plays two roles. As speakers, they try to make their speech as clear as they can. As listeners, they provide feedback to other group members by asking for repetitions if they have not heard or understood the other person's comment.

A few minutes are spent reviewing the targeted strategies while the entire group chorally practices each strategy in simple sentences as a warm-up. For example, the group is provided with a handout instructing them to take a deep breath and say loudly, "I am loud," as they exhale, then to slow their speech rate and say, "I take my time." To complete the warm-up, the coordinator leads a quick run-through of oral motor exercises.

The group then moves on to activities designed to encourage conversational interaction among the partici-

pants. These activities are the main focus of the session. They can take the forms of discussions of particular topics, having the participants ask each other questions to get to know each other better, or playing games—anything that requires the participants to communicate at least on the sentence level. Some activities that we have used are these:

- Current events: Discussions may focus on politics, weather, crime, movies, soap operas, or television shows.

- Hypothetical situations: Each participant is given a hypothetical situation and must say what he or she would do in the situation. Other members react to the answer.

- Opinions: Each participant is given a controversial topic or person, states his or her own opinion, and then the group discusses it.

- Autobiographical topics: A topic is chosen, such as family, friends, vacations, homes, grandchildren, weddings, or strokes, and each participant shares information or thoughts on the topic.

- Advice columns: Letters to advice columns are read, and the participants say how they would advise the individual. Their advice is compared to the "expert's."

- Barrier games: The group plays 20 Questions, Scruples, and Trivial Pursuit, among others.

Name	Goals	Cues	Comments
		.	

FIGURE 17-3.

Burke Rehabilitation Hospital Speech-Language and Audiology Worksheet for Dysarthria Group Coordinator. This worksheet can be used to organize all relevant information about the participants and their goals on one page (two for large groups). The coordinator can see at a glance which techniques a patient should be focusing on and record performance without flipping through the individual Referral Sheet/Report.

The coordinator facilitates the activities as necessary but encourages participants to do most of the talking and to be critical listeners, providing feedback when they have not heard or understood someone's comment. If a member is having particular difficulty using a strategy, the coordinator may solicit suggestions from other group members or may provide some direct intervention in the form of modeling, visual, or tactile cues in addition to the verbal feedback. If the group seems shy about providing feedback, the coordinator encourages it by modeling and by directly querying group members (e.g., "Mr. Smith, did you hear that?" or "Mrs. Jones, could you understand what she said?"). After one or two such queries, the participants usually feel more comfortable about letting each other know when a message has not gotten across. They also begin to provide positive feedback when the individual who has trouble with a strategy begins to use it successfully. The coordinator also acts as a facilitator to ensure that one or two people do not monopolize the discussion and to draw out individuals who are not spontaneously participating.

The coordinator keeps track of each participant's performance, either on the Referral Sheet/Report (see Figure 17-1) or on the Worksheet for Group Coordinator (Figure 17-3). The worksheet can be helpful because it has the information about all participants organized on one page. Its disadvantage is the time required to copy the relevant information for each patient onto the worksheet

and transfer it onto the Referral Sheet/Report. Therefore, use of the worksheet is optional.

Discharge Criteria

Inpatients are discharged from the group when one or more of the following criteria are met:

- The person is using the techniques successfully at least 80% of the time without cueing.

- The person elects to stop attending the group.

- The person's behavior disrupts the group or causes the other participants discomfort. Such individuals may be readmitted to the group if their cognitive or pragmatic abilities improve to the extent that their behavior becomes less disruptive.

- The individual is discharged from the inpatient hospital.

Reimbursement Issues

The hospital charges the inpatients a per diem rate, which is negotiated with the medical insurance carriers. This rate covers all services provided during the patient's stay, including the dysarthria group. The hospital keeps track of its actual expenses by using daily charge slips, which clinicians complete for each patient who attends the group. The fees used to track expenses are established by taking into account the clinician's time and salary, overhead costs, and average group size.

INPATIENT ORAL MOTOR GROUP

Philosophy of Program

The inpatient oral motor group was established so that we could provide instruction and feedback to dysarthric patients who needed to work on improving oral movements, maximum phonation time, or saliva management, without taking time during their individual treatment sessions to do so. The patients are expected to perform the exercises independently on a daily basis. The group allows us to ascertain whether they perform the exercises accurately, to monitor improvement in strength and range of motion, and to advance patients in the exercise regime as they improve.

Staff speech-language pathologists run these groups in our setting. If a state's licensure laws permit use of speech-language pathology assistants, however, they could probably run an oral motor group effectively, provided that the supervising speech-language pathologist (or the patient's primary clinician) reassesses the patient's oral motor performance periodically and prescribes changes in the exercises as the patient progresses.

Entry Criteria

Candidates for this group are inpatients whose performance during the assessment reveals reduced range of motion or weakness against resistance for the lips or tongue, whose maximum phonation time is inadequate to support connected speech, who have difficulty managing their saliva, or who need to work on using compensatory strategies at a word or sentence level. If a patient has aphasia in addition to dysarthria, the primary clinician and the group coordinator confer to determine whether the patient's language abilities are good enough to allow him or her to benefit from the group experience.

Assessment

The assessments are done individually, as described earlier, in Inpatient Dysarthria Groups, Assessment. People are referred to this group when the assessment reveals that they meet the entry criteria for the group. Because we run two oral motor groups, we can assign individuals to the groups based on the severity of their impairment. That is, one group can serve severely impaired people, whereas the other can include people with mild or moderate impairments.

Treatment Goals

The goals for the group are to use structured exercises to do the following:

- Increase range of motion and improve strength against resistance of the lips, jaw, and tongue through structured exercises
- Increase maximum phonation time
- Improve saliva management
- Improve speech intelligibility on the word and sentence level through compensatory strategies

Because the patients may be at different levels of performance in these areas, each patient has specific individualized goals within the scope of the broader group goals. The primary clinician uses the Oral Motor Group form (Figure 17-4) to make the referral to the group and to specify individual goals.

Documentation of Progress

The Oral Motor Group form serves as the basis for documenting progress. The group coordinator fills in information about the individual's performance, and the primary clinician uses this information to focus individual treatment. The information is also included in the weekly progress note.

Clinical Techniques

The group meets twice a week for 30-minute sessions. Group size varies from two to five individuals. Because members of the group may vary as patients are admitted and discharged, the session begins with introductions. The group members introduce themselves, using compensatory speech strategies that they've been practicing in their individual sessions. As in the dysarthria group, the session begins with a review of the group's purpose. The clinician emphasizes that, in addition to practicing their exercises and speech strategies, each member also serves as a listener who can provide feedback to the other members about how well they use their speech strategies and as an observer who can provide feedback about performance of exercises.

The group practices range-of-motion exercises for the jaw, lips, and tongue. Mirrors are available for individuals who need visual feedback. With the clinician explaining and demonstrating as they go, the group practices jaw opening and closing, lip puckering and retraction, tongue protrusion, tongue lateralization, tongue elevation, and tongue depression exercises. The group is reminded to try to keep the movements symmetric and to try to reach

Name: _____   Room: _____

Speech-language pathologist: _____

Goals: (indicate assistance level as needed)	Week 1	Week 2	Week 3
_____ Perform oral motor exercises Status:			
_____ Increase maximum phonation time Status:			
_____ Improve saliva management Status:			
_____ Use compensatory speech strategies List:			

FIGURE 17-4.

Burke Rehabilitation Hospital Speech-Language and Audiology Oral Motor Group form. This form serves as a referral sheet and documentation of a person's performance. The primary clinician specifies the goals when the referral is made. The clinician who leads the group notes the patient's performance weekly under the appropriate columns and writes comments under each goal if necessary.

their maximum range of motion and then hold the stretch before relaxing. The clinician provides verbal feedback and tactile cueing as necessary. People who need to start at the level of passive range of motion are shown how to assist the muscle movements. Each exercise is repeated ten times before proceeding to the next exercise.

Resistance is then added to the exercises by handing out tongue depressors and demonstrating how to use them to resist the movements of the lips and tongue. The clinician checks on techniques and provides feedback to improve performance as necessary.

Next, maximum phonation time is addressed. Using a clock with a second hand or a stopwatch that all the members can see, the clinician instructs them to take a deep breath and to say "ah" on the exhalation. They should make their voice last as long as they can by watching the clock or stopwatch. The clinician usually provides them with goals that get increasingly longer on each attempt (e.g., first for 3 seconds, then 5 seconds, then 7 seconds), working up to phonation that lasts 15–20 seconds as individuals improve.

The next set of exercises focuses on rapidly alternating speech movements (e.g., "puh," "tuh," "kuh," "puhtuhkuh," or some variation). Depending on the group's level of per-

formance, word or sentence drills chosen to target specific phonemes that are problematic for the individuals may also be addressed. These are usually performed chorally with reminders to the members to use their speech strategies. Feedback is provided as necessary.

To improve saliva management, members are guided in achieving and maintaining lip closure for progressively longer periods. A timer is set and reset during the session to remind the people working on this goal to swallow at least as often as the timer goes off.

Discharge Criteria

The discharge criteria are essentially the same as those for the inpatient dysarthria group.

Reimbursement Issues

Reimbursement issues are the same as those for the inpatient dysarthria group.

OUTPATIENT DYSARTHRIA GROUPS

Philosophy of Program

The philosophy of the outpatient dysarthria groups is similar to that of the inpatient dysarthria group. People are usually referred to a group when they have maximized their progress in individual treatment but continue to have difficulty generalizing this progress to spontaneous conversational situations. Each group is established for a set number of weeks. At the end of that time, members are discharged or referred into another group, if that is an appropriate option. Typically, the groups are established for patients who need to generalize newly acquired techniques to conversational situations. However, we have also had groups that we have established at the request of the local Parkinson support group, for example, which are designed to address the speech problems of that specific impairment.

Entry Criteria

Entry criteria for outpatient groups differ depending on the specific goals of the group that is being formed. For example, the group that we formed at the request of the Parkinson support group included any member of the support group who wanted to participate. Usually, we try to build groups with members who are similar in terms of severity of speech impairment, goals, and age.

Assessment and Treatment Goals

In general, candidates for the group are assessed individually, so that each patient can establish individual goals. Sometimes, however, as in the case of the group started for the Parkinson support group, no individual assessments are done, and goals are established for the group as a whole.

Documentation of Progress

Forms similar to those used with the inpatient groups are used to outline individual goals and record progress. Information from these forms is used for documentation in progress notes and in discharge summaries.

Clinical Techniques

The techniques used in these groups are similar to those used in the inpatient groups. Because a time limit is imposed on the number of sessions, however, we typically try to emphasize one goal or strategy per week. For example, because the members of the Parkinson support group had not had speech therapy in a while, the speech groups began with a short discussion about each goal or strategy as a review. They then used exercises or other activities to allow the patients to practice the strategy while the clinician provided feedback and suggestions for continuing

the work at home. One week might focus on respiration, the next on phonation, the third on pacing, the fourth on articulation, and so forth. The members were expected to incorporate strategies from the previous weeks as the sessions progressed.

Discharge Criteria

Because we make it clear from the outset that the group will meet for only a set number of weeks, the members understand that, at the end of that time, they will be discharged from the group. If a patient is continuing to have difficulty generalizing the techniques at the end of a group, we may refer that patient into another group if an appropriate one exists or is about to be formed.

Reimbursement Issues

In our experience, most insurance plans do not reimburse for group treatment. We make it clear to the patients at the outset that they must pay for the group themselves. We work with the hospital's business office to determine fees for the groups. The fees are determined by taking into account the clinician's time and salary, overhead costs for the space and supplies, and the number of people who will be part of the group. To avoid the problems that can occur when space and clinician hours are set aside for the group but group members start dropping out, it's often easiest to charge one fee at the start to cover all sessions. It is made clear to members that because the hospital's expenses must be covered, the fee is not refundable if they miss sessions. Naturally, exceptions can be made for unusual circumstances on a case-by-case basis, if necessary.

CLINICIAN AND PATIENT RESPONSES TO THE GROUPS

Speech-language pathologists have been pleased with the outcomes of the groups. The dysarthria groups have allowed us to spend time specifically focusing on generalization-promoting techniques in ways that are not possible in individual sessions. The oral motor group has allowed us to provide supervised time for oral motor exercises without using individual speech treatment time for the purpose. Feedback about the patients' group performance has been valuable in helping us to refine our work with them in individual sessions.

More important, patients' responses to the groups have been very positive. Mr. I., one of our inpatients, said, "One of the benefits we get out of the group is the review of our speaking strategies and techniques. But I think what's even more important than that is that we have the opportunity to speak spontaneously, as we talk to one another, and I think that's beneficial." Sometimes our inpatients are resistant to attending the group at first because they are self-conscious about their impaired intelligibility. Mrs. M. was one such patient. After a few sessions, she told us,

> I didn't want to come (to the group) because I couldn't speak at all when I came in, and I felt very self-conscious, but I came anyway. And I found out that I could speak with some other people and that they did help me. And I think that I benefit by this group along with individual therapy. I think it's a whole package that I need, that I didn't want, but I did want it after I came here.

One of our outpatients, Mrs. R., who was in a group after the completion of her individual therapy sessions, also felt that the group sessions enhanced the gains she had made in individual therapy. She said, "I took private sessions first and that was very helpful, and then when I came to the group I found that it is very good for me at this point in time. The individual work was perfect for the beginning, but I think this group is helping me more now."

Patients have provided similar positive feedback about our oral motor groups. Many patients are sensitive about the changes in facial symmetry and saliva control caused by their strokes. Several patients reported that they found it comforting to work on improving their oral motor abilities in the presence of others who were experiencing similar impairment of function. The group created a fun, interactive setting for practicing their exercise programs.

In summary, clinicians and patients agree that groups have been useful adjuncts to individual treatment for dysarthria. Groups require special skills of clinicians: organizing and tracking the goals of individual patients in the session, facilitating spontaneous interactions in a semi-structured setting, and knowing when to intervene and when to sit back and watch. Similarly, groups pose special challenges to patients. In a group, they must overcome their self-consciousness about facial asymmetry or less-than-perfect speech, applying strategies from individual sessions to the sometimes fast-moving conversational interactions. They must also act as a deputized clinician to help other group members with motivation, feedback, and tips. When clinicians and patients meet these challenges, we all benefit.

Acknowledgments
The authors would like to acknowledge Caroline Bak Bossinas, Shari Strikowsky Harvey, Jennifer O'Hare, Karen Juliano, Judite Pedro, Laura Reese, Michelle Renz, Andrea Sieger, and Barbara Yau for their valuable contributions to the dysarthria groups. We also acknowledge the many dysarthric individuals who have participated in our groups. We learn at least as much from them as they do from us.

REFERENCES

1. Stokes TF, Baer DM. An implicit technology of generalization. J Appl Behav Anal 1977;10:349–367.
2. Berry W, Sanders S. Environmental Education: The Universal Management Approach for Adults with Dysarthria. In W Berry (ed), Clinical Dysarthria. San Diego: College Hill Press, 1983;203–216.
3. Sullivan MD, Brune PJ, Beukelman DR. Maintenance of Speech Changes following Group Treatment for Hypokinetic Dysarthria of Parkinson's Disease. In DA Robin, KM York, DR Beukelman (eds), Disorders of Motor Speech: Assessment, Treatment, and Clinical Characterization. Baltimore: Paul H. Brookes, 1996;287–307.

Index